MASSAGE FOR A
PEACEFUL PREGNANCY

Massage
for a *peaceful pregnancy*

A Daily Book
for New Mothers and Fathers

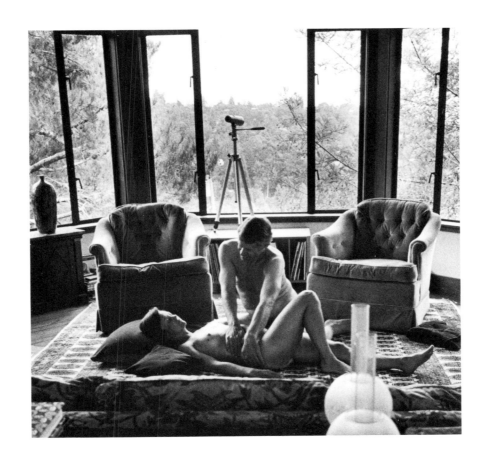

Written and Photographed
by Gordon Inkeles

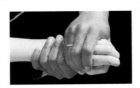

AN ARCATA ARTS BOOK

An Arcata Arts Book
P.O.B. 800, Bayside, CA. 95524
gi@arcata-arts.com
http://arcata-arts.com

ISBN – 10: 0-9748535-4-2
ISBN – 13: 978-0-9748535-4-3

Library of Congress Control Number:
2006909418

First Perigee printing 1984
First Arcata Arts printing March 2007

The author wishes to express appreciation for permission to quote and reproduce artwork from Sigga Bjornsson and Felicia Trujillo.

Book design by Jon Goodchild/Triad
Cover design by Rama Wong
Cover art by Sigga Bjornsson
Cover consultant: Molly Maguire
Art Director: Iris Schencke
Special Thanks: David Hodge, Matt Inkeles

Printed in China

Always consult a doctor if you are in doubt about a medical condition, and observe the cautions given in this book.

for Iris
because you were there
you touched it

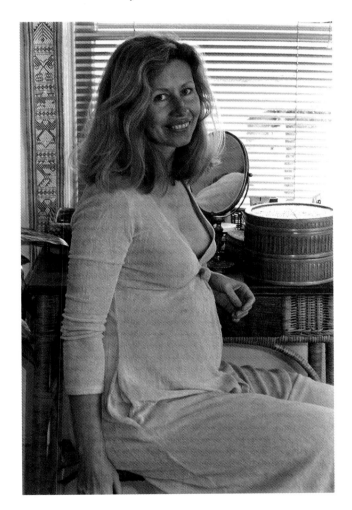

Contents

4. A Complete Head Massage

5. Late Pregnancy

6. A Complete Back Massage

7. The Birth

8. After the Birth

9. Specialized Massage

To the Expectant Father

This book is mainly for you.

If you are preparing to be a father for the first time, you probably feel confused about exactly what your role is supposed to be. Looking through a typical pregnancy book, you may have found a few words of advice: "Be loving and supportive," or "Be understanding when her moods change suddenly." That's comforting to know, but what are you supposed to *do*? Should you take charge of keeping everyone cheerful no matter how you feel? Or should you remain in the background, tiptoeing uselessly around the woman you love during the time of your greatest shared experience? As the pregnancy progresses and a woman requires special kinds of attention, your role can become more confusing. You recognize that many women become lonely and alienated in the final trimester, when radical body changes take place. And you know that pregnant women get little compassion from men who have been conditioned to give up on touching once sex has become difficult. You are committed and want a different role for yourself. What can you do on a daily basis for the next nine months that will help?

The massage solution lets you deal with the body as it is, not as it could be. During a time of such rapid change, your partner needs to know that you accept her. If you don't make that clear she may become like the athlete, familiar to all sports masseurs, who feels guilty for injuring a perfect body and needing a massage. Many pregnant women experience the same sort of guilt simply because they need support, but are afraid to ask for it. They begin to see pregnancy as a difficult period during which a woman becomes a terrible burden on friends and family.

There is no better time to change this negative self-image than during a massage. You become directly involved with your partner, using your own two hands. She can *feel* that you care because during a massage nothing is more important to you than her well-being. Experiencing an hour of continuous physical pleasure is tangible proof of your affection and a powerful antidote to the guilt habit. Learning to give pleasure with your hands will bring peace to a woman throughout pregnancy and at the birth itself. Pregnancy offers a father the opportunity to learn massage techniques that can be shared and will eventually become an important part of family life.

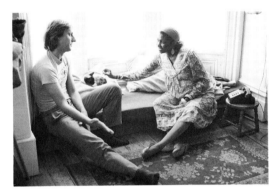

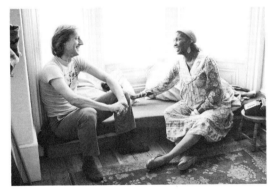

To the Expectant Mother

Your role during massage is to do as little as possible. This is a time for you to relax, enjoy being cared for, and become familiar with your changing body. Along with the obvious emotional treasures that regular massage offers expectant parents, there are important physical benefits for a woman. Headaches, back problems, neck and shoulder pain, cramps, constipation, fatigue, and nervous tension can be reduced or eliminated. Massage improves circulation to every part of the body, particularly to the legs, where varicosities may be prevented. Cramp-induced muscle spasms as well as a wide range of stress-related illnesses are likely to disappear. If staying away from unnecessary drugs is part of your health plan during pregnancy, massage will show you a way to eliminate most over-the-counter medication. After the birth, massage will elevate your mood and erase or reduce the visible effects of stretching of the breasts, stomach, and torso. It will relieve pressures in the breasts that can block lactation and, finally, bring peace and happiness to your new baby.

A full body massage offers you one hour of uninterrupted pleasure. Your partner does all the work; you do nothing at all.

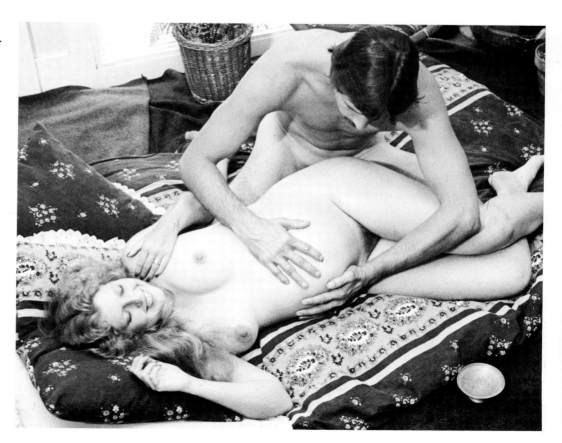

Like yoga and dance, massage has its own aesthetic. People look a certain way when they are being massaged. Their eyes remain closed, and as conscious posing becomes impossible the still, poised look of a dancer who has achieved a perfect sense of balance sometimes emerges. Deer standing quietly in a winter forest convey the same impression of serene repose. Unfortunately the published images of pregnant women have not always met this ideal of loveliness. Pregnancy is still photographed either as a grotesque, terribly awkward ordeal or as a gauzy, out-of-focus little girl's dream. This book offers another image of pregnancy, one that is thousands of years old. Here is the pregnant woman as sensualist, using her body, enjoying it, and enjoying being touched. In these unposed pictures you begin to recognize the grace and peace of the dancer as she relaxes and surrenders to massage. This is the way massage actually looks, uncomplicated but full of rare surprise.

For many years *Gray's Anatomy* and a host of imitators have presented the human body as an inert, desiccated place, where tissues are routinely sliced in half to expose internal structures. This is the surgeon's, not the masseur's, reality. Split a tree down the middle, and you reveal its inner workings, only to lose the sense of what it was as a tree. The two women who illustrated this book managed to peer inside the body and find systems you can touch during massage while ensuring that the drawings continue to look real and human. Felicia Trujillo did the diagrams of internal body changes and the elegant "Nerves of the Back" drawing on page 111. The amazing Sigga Bjornsson transformed the women who actually appear in this book into classic anatomical illustrations. These women present the body as a masseur must see it: The surface lymphatic system is separated from the interior one, the exposed arteries are identified, and the muscles that support the head are set apart.

Pregnancy has touched the lives of almost everyone involved with this project, and twice, while I postponed the photography hoping for better light conditions, one of the models gave birth. Jon Goodchild, designer of *The Art of Sensual Massage* and *The New Massage,* chose a softer design for this book to complement its theme. He appears with his pregnant wife on the cover. Diane Reverand, the Putnam editor who watched over *Massage and Peaceful Pregnancy* from conception to birth, gave birth to a baby boy the day the manuscript arrived in New York.

Gordon Inkeles,
San Francisco, *October 1983*

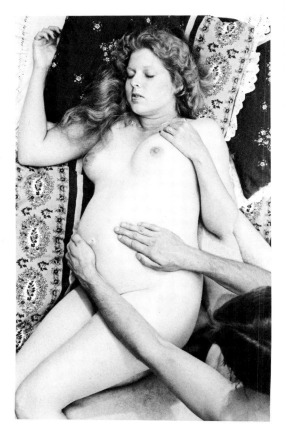

Photographing pregnancy is a question of timing and the hesitant photographer can expect to pay the ultimate price. I am most grateful to the patient couples who presented a new reality for my inquisitive lens nearly every week. This book does not offer a peek inside the womb at the developing fetus or a ringside seat at a birth. We must be content with surfaces in massage; I left the fetuses to their private world and the parents to theirs.

Notes on the New Edition

On a brilliant San Francisco afternoon one year after this book originally appeared, my son Matthew was born. I did the easy part: nineteen hours of massage, which I applied during the contractions. My wife Iris did the hard part: the nineteen hours of labor itself.

When I say the massage was "easy" I'm not really exaggerating. No great strength or endurance is needed to do massage; it's as easy as walking down the street. Indeed, I was grateful to have something helpful to do with my hands during the labor. Having put to good use the techniques described in these pages for our entire pregnancy, I had plenty of practice. By the time our son was born I felt connected to the birth process in unexpected ways.

Like all parents, my wife and I occasionally relive the first moments of our child's life, I can remember holding my son for the first time a few minutes after he was born. I saw his eyes focus on mine with a peculiar intensity that I'll never forget.

But we also connected on a tactile level, because as I began stroking his tiny back, just minutes after he entered this world, our first massage began. In the months to come, as massage became part of Matt's bathing routine and a favorite moment for all, I became acquainted with his precious smile.

During our nine months of pregnancy we both learned that massage seldom disappoints; the blissful expressions you see in this book are real, not posed: no machines or medications were needed. After Matt was born we continued with massage. Twenty-one years later we're still at it.

Now, dear reader, it's your turn. As an expectant father, you are about to embark on one of life's crowning experiences: the birth of your child. Whether you are called upon to do massage at the birth or not, (see p. 120) massage will become a shared pleasure that will bring your family closer together.

Think of the techniques in this book as a gift for your partner and your newborn child. And bring them both home smiling.

Gordon Inkeles

Bayside, California
January 2007

MASSAGE FOR A
PEACEFUL PREGNANCY

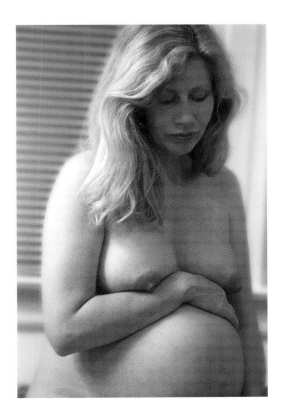

A ship under sail and
a big bellied woman are
the handsomest things
that can be seen common.

Benjamin Franklin

PREPARING
TO DO MASSAGE

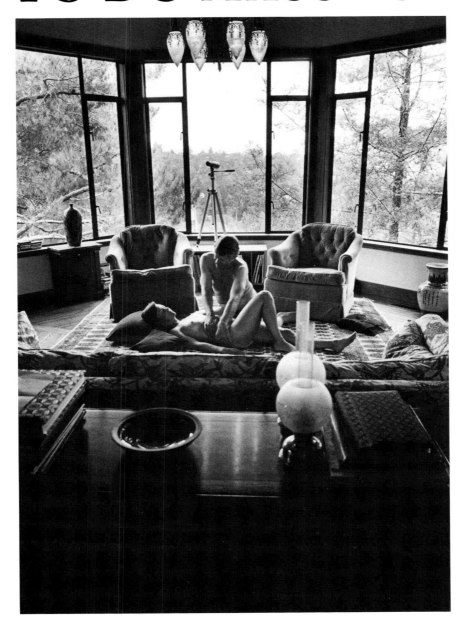

A First Massage

. . . time, hurry, doing, did not
exist, the accumulating seconds and
minutes and hours to which in its
well state the body is slave both
waking and sleeping, now reversed
and time now the lip-server and
mendicant to the body's pleasure
instead of the body thrall to time's
headlong course.

William Faulkner

At its best, a first massage can be the sort of experience your partner will remember for the rest of her
life. People who have never experienced real massage are amazed to discover how wonderful they
feel after an hour of kneading, stroking, and circulation movements. Even just a few *minutes* spent
working on a headache can eliminate intense throbbing that has persisted all day. That's one of the
things human hands can do: ease pain. People begin
to understand this all at once after a first massage,
and you're likely to be nearby when the realization
hits. It's an intoxicating moment, one that can be
repeated with each massage.

Once you've selected a massage area and established the right sort of mood, think carefully about
your partner's senses, and do everything possible to
please them. All your final preparation should center on this idea: What will she experience while
you're massaging; what will she actually feel?

Since the experience is new and very special,
it's a good idea to take a few extra minutes preparing yourself and your environment. Think about
how much time you spent getting ready for your
last dinner party. A meal is consumed, enjoyed, and
then forgotten, but a first massage will be
remembered.

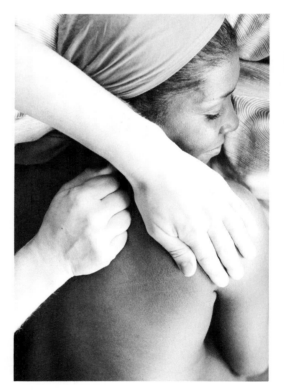

Inside the body muscular, glandular
and vascular systems are
stimulated. Lymphatic flow
increases and the nerves are
soothed. There isn't a single organ
in the body which doesn't benefit
from massage.

You can do massage in any house or
apartment. Set up outdoors on a
warm summer evening. No specialized equipment or highly technical
training is necessary.

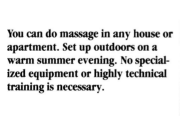

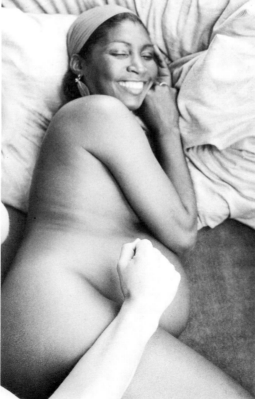

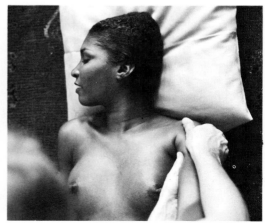

Choosing a Massage Area

Before you begin massaging, it's always useful to consider briefly how your massage area is going to feel to a pregnant woman. A few minutes spent creating the right kind of atmosphere will convince your partner, the moment she steps into the room, that something very special is about to happen. She's going to experience massage with her eyes closed, and this will automatically intensify all the other senses. An intensified awareness of scent, taste, sound, and, of course, touch will help her enjoy the massage that is about to begin. You can provide something interesting for each one of the senses all the way through a massage. A pleasant taste will linger for a long time. So many memories are tied to characteristic scent. Why not give her something special to remember during her massage? Just one stick of incense will scent a room for more than an hour; choose one your partner likes, or you may prefer to scent your massage oil with a few drops of her favorite perfume or essence. If you live in an apartment, it may not be possible to control

every sound that passes through the walls, but you can easily substitute your own. More on that later.

Before a first massage, most pregnant women have absolutely no idea what to expect and may seem very nervous. Any effort you make to create the best possible mood in your massage area will help your partner relax and surrender to an hour or two of uninterrupted pleasure. The place where you decide to do massage should be warm, comfortable, and pleasant. If you appear organized and confident, she will settle down quickly and begin to relax.

A massage begins with your partner lying down before you, eyes closed and totally naked. Above all, she must trust you not to do *anything* that would be painful. One moment of pain can destroy an hour of blissful massage work. Pain not only ruins a massage but violates her trust in you. Massage is pleasure—uninterrupted pleasure.

No matter how skillful your technique, the entire massage will fail if your partner gets chilled. You must arrange to keep the massage surface at

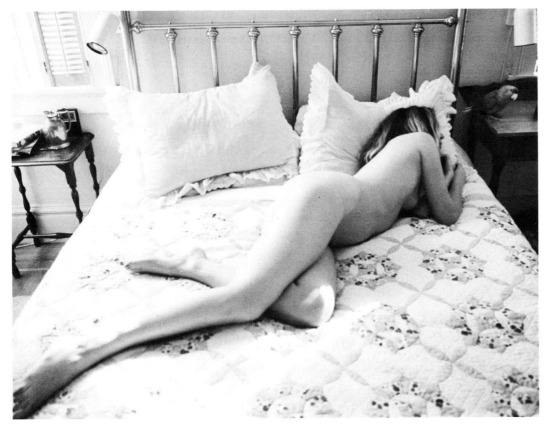

Find a firm surface for massage; a very soft mattress just won't do. Four inches of foam rubber will support your partner nicely, as will large pillows or a couple of sleeping bags covered with sheets and towels. You'll need to give your partner room to rearrange herself, particularly if she's in her third trimester. And of course, you will need room to move around her while you're massaging.

seventy-five degrees Fahrenheit for several hours so your partner will be warm during the massage and for some time afterward. If you live in a cold climate, temperature control of the massage surface is particularly important, and it will probably be necessary to heat the entire room to a temperature higher than seventy-five degrees. You may work up a sweat during the massage, but your partner, whose metabolism slows down as you relax her, will remain perfectly comfortable.

See if you can arrange everything so that there will be no interruptions during the massage. Of course, that's not always possible. If you are interrupted, try to keep touching your partner while you deal with an unexpected knock on the door or a cat that slipped in through an open window. Massage is contact; make it last.

Low lights, soft music and a harmonious atmosphere will begin to relax your partner before you start massaging. Sometimes massage works best in an unused part of your home.

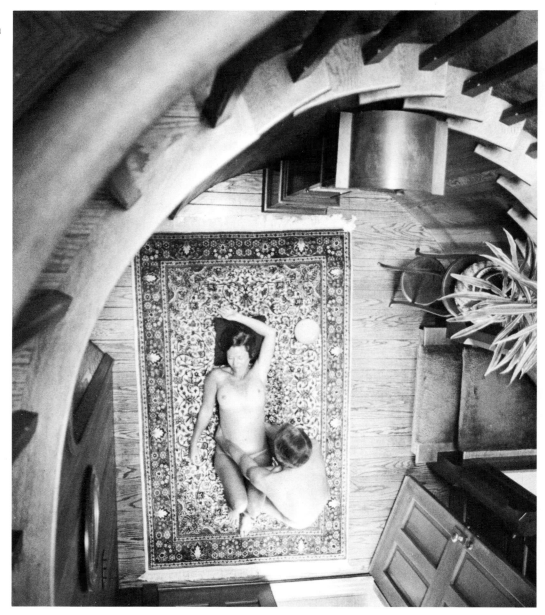

Oil

Most women have enjoyed the naturally resilient feeling of oiled skin, but since the oil was self-applied, they missed the pleasure of being stroked by somebody else. A first massage can serve as an introduction to a host of new feelings, among them the delicious sensation you get when warm oil is spread across your body by another human being. Oiling is part of massage and should never be viewed as a separate process. You'll find ways to combine stroking oil onto your partner with specific massage movements. More on that when we get into massaging.

Oil lubricates the skin and will be used everywhere on the body except the scalp. You don't need to bother with overpriced "commercial" preparations when most light clear vegetable oils (like coconut or almond) will do as well. You may want to scent the oil with fresh lemon, which is very good for the skin, or with your partner's favorite perfume. It's very important to choose a scent that pleases her because by the end of a massage nearly every part of her body will be oiled. Be careful not to overscent; a few drops are all you need for eight ounces of clear oil.

Almost any container for the oil will do, but remember that even the most experienced masseur can easily knock over a cup or bowl. A small plastic squeeze bottle will eliminate this problem, particularly if it's the kind with a built-in shutoff valve. Empty shampoo bottles can easily be washed out and refilled with massage oil. If you live in a hot climate, you might want to refrigerate your oil between massages. It takes only one minute to warm a few ounces of oil in a microwave oven; a few minutes more in a pot of boiling water.

In fact, unless you live in a tropical climate, it's best to use heated oil. While you're massaging, your partner's metabolism will slow down, leaving her very sensitive to temperature changes. Cold oil will shock her and destroy the relaxed mood you're working to create. Heat your oil for a few minutes before you begin until it's almost hot to the touch and you won't need to warm it again while you're massaging.

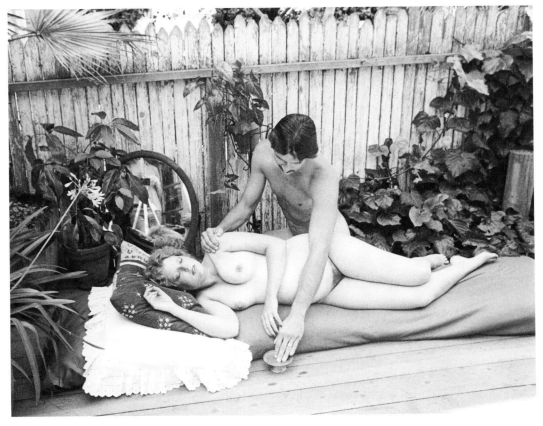

Put the oil where it can be reached easily while you're massaging. Take it with you when you move from one part of your partner's body to another but remember not to break contact when the oil is moved.

Sound

The acute awareness your partner develops the moment she closes her eyes makes her very sensitive to any sounds that reach the massage area. Listen carefully, and you will hear what she hears. A "quiet" party next door suddenly becomes very loud, a television set several rooms away chatters on, and street traffic begins to seem terribly intrusive. Even if you could eliminate all these sounds, there remains the bane of every serious masseur: appliance noise. Most people take no notice of a refrigerator, dishwasher, or washing machine as it cycles on and off. Unfortunately these sounds can come crashing in on your partner just as she is beginning to relax. This is not to suggest that a refrigerator must be disconnected before a massage, but you can eliminate all kinds of unpleasant sounds by simply substituting music for random noise. Choose something quiet and relaxed that will appeal to your partner. Continuous music radio stations, a cassette recorder with automatic reverse, or a record changer will allow you to forget about adjusting the music once it has begun. Music can begin to set the right mood even before you begin

Choose your massage music carefully because fetal activity is directly influenced by external sounds. Loud rhythmic music will agitate the fetus and speed up the tempo of your massage; a quiet lyrical piece has the reverse effect.

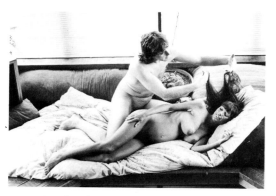

massaging, but there is one other alternative that can be very interesting, and if you're lucky enough to find the right conditions, you may wish to explore it: silence.

In a perfectly silent environment it's not necessary to add music unless your partner asks for it. Massage itself has a sound, and since every movement is rhythmic, the sound is syncopated. It varies from body to body. If all other sounds are eliminated, this one becomes quietly hypnotic. Muted and very far away you may recognize something like the sound of water running over smooth stones, a flock of starlings passing overhead, dry leaves rustling in the wind; what you are actually

hearing is the sound of skin against skin, oil rippling across the body, and hair being brushed gently. Silently your partner shares these sounds with you. When was the last time she listened to her hair being combed?

Wind, water, breath, and sigh—these are the natural sounds of human beings touching and caring for one another. They are as much a part of human life, and certainly far more ancient than, any kind of music. A confident masseur can orchestrate the sounds of various strokes and make them a part of the massage experience. To be effective, simple kneading requires more patience than technique. Once you have learned how to use the thumbs properly, your hands open and close effortlessly as they move back and forth over a part of your partner's body. If the movement is going to be repeated forty or fifty times, it is finally the *sound* that one concentrates on while the hands continue patiently in rhythm. Listen closely while kneading the larger muscle groups, and you may recognize something very close to the sound of small waves breaking on a forgotten beach.

People who automatically reach for the radio whenever things grow quiet find an unexpected surprise in massage. They learn to experience stillness without panicking and escape, for a while, from background noise that only masks reality. The soft, rhythmic sounds of massage have a hypnotic quality that helps both the masseur and his partner; repetition comes easily to the masseur who listens to the sound of his work, while the steady rhythms relax a woman almost immediately.

A Massage Plan

Put your oil and towels within reach so you won't have to interrupt the massage to search for them. It's always helpful to decide which parts of the body you're going to massage and arrange yourself and your partner so you can reach them easily. If you're working with the side lying position in one of the later trimesters (see pages 86–87), you'll need extra pillows to keep your partner comfortable. You may decide to massage the whole left side of the body from foot to head and then, after finishing the head, descend along the torso and leg to the right foot. Sometimes it's fun to massage each foot, each leg, each arm, the torso, and then the head. That approach will require moving about a bit more, but for the sake of variation and symmetry, you may want to try it.

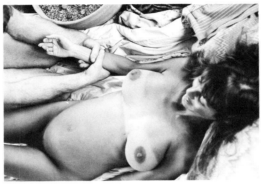

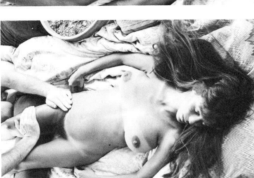

Remove ticking clocks, that become remarkably loud and invasive, from your massage area. Clocks are useless during massage because the experience can't be rushed.

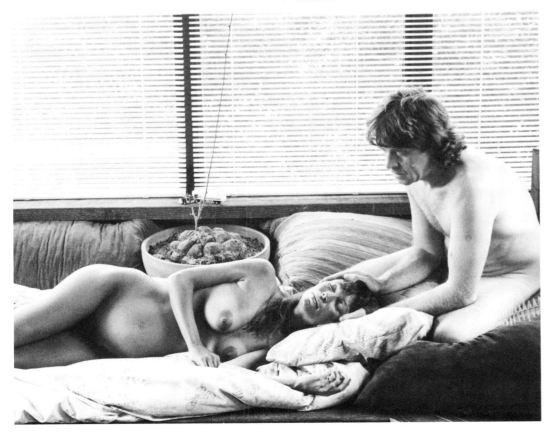

If you're massaging near a window adjust the curtains or blinds so you and your partner won't suddenly be roasted by the afternoon sun. Choose an evenly heated place with no drafts.

23

What Feels Good . . . And What Doesn't

Remain calm, when interrupted, and try to maintain contact. When your partner settles down, continue with what you were doing as though nothing had happened. In a few moments the interruption will be forgotten; during massage your partner lives entirely in her body.

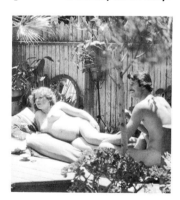

Do

Keep your fingers together when you knead and stroke. During kneading let one hand go all the way to the open position while the other moves in to pick up a bit of flesh between the thumb and opposing fingers.

Stay in physical contact with your partner whenever you have to stop massaging for any reason. Be sure to do this whether you're moving from one side of the body to the other or stopping for a sip of water.

Keep all your movements smooth and rhythmic. Strokes should blend into each other until, finally, what your partner *feels* is one long continuous movement up and down her body.

Use just enough oil to make stroking easy. Go ahead and add more as oil is absorbed by her skin and your hands.

Be attentive to your partner throughout a massage. There are many nonverbal cues that will indicate approval or disapproval. Sighs and moans mean that she likes what you're doing and would appreciate more of the same. Stop immediately if something you do becomes unpleasant for her, and go on to the next movement.

Pay attention to the small details of your partner's body, particularly at the end of long movements. Include the tops of her shoulders and the sides of her hips when you stroke up the arms and legs.

Establish a rhythm at the beginning of the massage and stay with it. Big strokes and little strokes move at the same speed.

Let your partner decide where pillows belong. Try to have several different sizes on hand.

Don't

Let your fingers drift apart into a webbed-foot position. With your fingers opened the stroke looses half its effectiveness. Your partner will feel the difference, and you will find it difficult to maintain a consistent rhythm.

Break contact the moment something comes up that surprises you. Into every massage a few specks of floor debris, sand, or grit may fall. Remove them from her body with one hand while you keep contact with the other.

Bear down too hard near a painful area. Avoid abrupt transitions and short scrubbing motions. You're massaging a woman, not waxing a floor. She will respond best to rhythmic circular movements.

Create oil slicks on her back, where any kind of concentrated work will become impossible. There should always be a tiny bit of friction between your hands and her skin. Don't, however, allow the friction to become so great that you begin tugging at her skin.

Encourage conversation. She'll let you know if part of her body needs more attention, but this isn't a good time to tell her the story of your life. Remember that some people will chatter compulsively because they are afraid of being touched. Too much talking will eventually come between your partner and her massage.

Forget a toe. The toe will feel hurt and abandoned.

Watch a clock while you're massaging. Don't try to fit a massage into a tight schedule between two high-pressure events. If your partner is leading a stressful life, massage her at the end of the day, and let her fall asleep afterward.

Allow her to become cold or uncomfortable. Never do anything that hurts your partner.

You should avoid any kind of massage if . . .

your partner has an infection or fever.
you can see extensive skin eruptions or bruises.
a doctor has advised against it.

Avoid massaging an area where your partner has a

- ☐ bruise.
- ☐ skin eruption.
- ☐ inflamed joint.
- ☐ sensitive vein(s).
- ☐ tumor.
- ☐ painful reaction.

Jewelry should come off before a massage begins, as should contact lenses if you plan to massage the eyes. Be sure to put these tiny goodies in a safe, easy-to-find place, lest the two of you end a massage on your hands and knees creeping around on the living room rug.

Testing the Massage Area

If you're beginning with massage in a new place, a good way to test the area is to put your partner in it and leave her alone for a while. Let her lie perfectly still and simply experience the place as it is. After a few minutes she'll be ready for some quiet talk about the things that matter most in massage. Most beds will make head and foot massage more difficult, but your partner may find a firm mattress more comfortable than any setup on the floor.

Is the room warm enough? Perhaps there's an open window you forgot to close. What sounds manage to penetrate to the massage area? What does she smell? Will extra pillows be necessary? Just before you begin massaging is the best time to discuss these questions and give her what she wants.

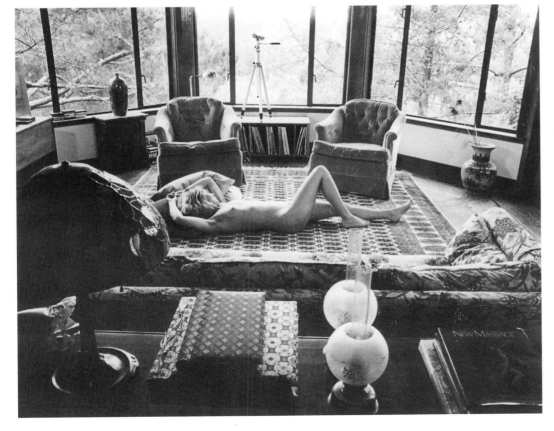

Most telephone answering machines will continue working when the phone is unplugged. A "do not disturb" sign on the front door alerts unexpected visitors. In the evening, one candle provides enough light for massage.

Setting Things Up

Are you expecting phone calls or guests?

Are children or pets likely to disturb you?

Is the massage *surface* at least seventy-five degrees, and will it stay that warm for the next few hours?

Are there any disturbing sounds or smells reaching the massage area?

Is the massage area comfortable for both of you, and is it clean?

Do you have various size pillows on hand?

Have you set up "extra" equipment which might be necessary if you want to burn incense or play massage music?

Will you be able to move easily all the way around your partner?

Final Preparations

Do you have enough warm oil on hand, and can it be reached easily?

Is the oil likely to spill while you're massaging?

Do you have plenty of clean towels?

Has she removed contact lenses and jewelry?

Are there any sensitive areas on her body that you might need to avoid?

Do you have a general massage plan?

Are you ready to be silent?

If it's your partner's first massage a little quiet talk at the outset sometimes helps to relax her. It's useful to explain that there is nothing painful or unpleasant in massage. Try to keep your comments brief and don't encourage a long conversation. This close to the massage the tone you use when speaking becomes very important.

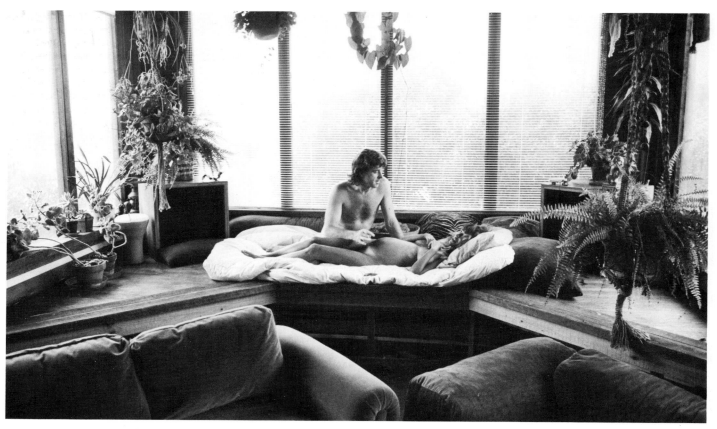

Making Contact

Begin touching your partner the moment she closes her eyes. You can choose any part of the body for your first contact; hand holding is particularly effective with pregnant women because it's gentle and familiar. Wherever you decide to touch her, it's important to remember that the massage itself has now begun. From this moment on you should continue touching your partner throughout the massage, even when you move from one part of the body to another. Breaking contact, just for a moment, will leave her feeling abandoned and interrupt the exquisitely peaceful mood you've been working to build. An experienced masseur with a 100-movement repertoire cannot afford to break contact for a moment. Doing so he will accomplish less than a beginner who hesitates constantly but remembers to stay with his partner while deciding what to do next.

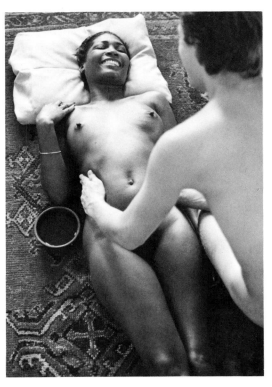

Some masseurs like to initiate contact by oiling the skin. With that approach your partner's first massage experience becomes the luxurious sensation of warm oil being spread across her body. Once again, most women have oiled themselves; few have been oiled by someone else.

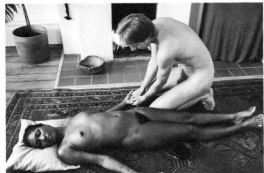

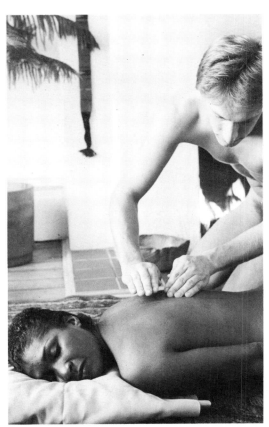

If you don't want to jump right into the massage and your partner is sensitive about being touched simply take her hand and hold it. Everyone is accustomed to being touched on the hands and the fingertips are one of the most tactile parts of the body. Remain still for a while and let her surrender to the feeling. Then, when everything is perfectly quiet, begin massaging her hands.

BASIC MASSAGE
FOR THE
WHOLE BODY

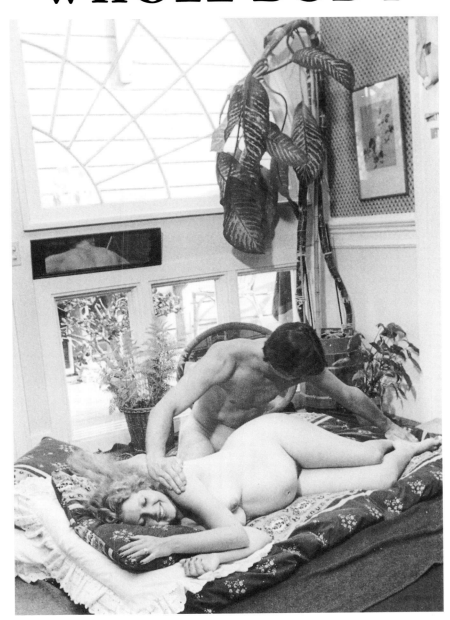

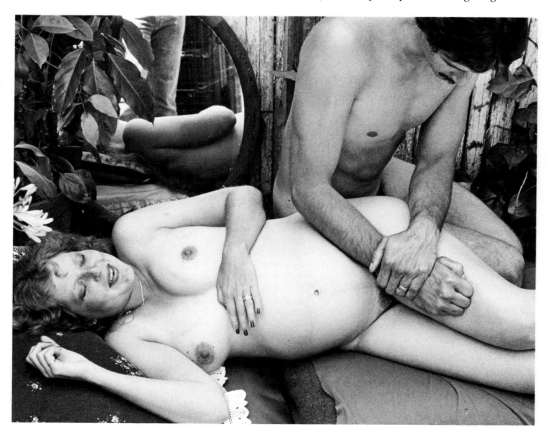

Introduction to Basic Massage

This stillness to which all returns, this is reality . . .

Peter Mathiessen

Start massaging around your partner's body as soon as you've learned a few movements. In the beginning, don't worry about fine anatomical details or perfect technique. All touch feels good and your partner will appreciate the continuous physical contact.

Massage for a Peaceful Pregnancy is organized around areas of the body that most need massage during the various stages of pregnancy. To that end the two major parts of the book, "Early Pregnancy" and "Late Pregnancy," are more useful guides for a masseur than the usual monthly or trimester divisions. Ideally a man will continue massaging his partner right through her pregnancy. Men who do will note that one day a woman can no longer lie comfortably on her stomach no matter how many pillows are added. The arrival of that day varies from woman to woman, but when it comes, late pregnancy has begun and she must recline on her side. A masseur is then confronted with entirely new body surfaces, and he needs to learn techniques which are designed for the special requirements of this time.

Late pregnancy also marks the point when physical stresses shift from the neck and shoulder area to the lower back. Do no more than massage those two parts of the body, and you will make a very real contribution to your partner's well-being and the health of your developing child. Of course,

if a woman enjoys your neck and shoulder massage, there is something more you can do for her—you can massage the rest of her body.

During massage the best way to relax any single part of the body is to relax all the other parts as well. Movements in this section, for instance, can be modified slightly and extended to include almost any part of the body. Throughout the book you will find ways to improvise on these basic strokes so they will fit the changing shape of a woman's body during pregnancy. Combine them later, when you become more comfortable massaging her, and create a basic but satisfying full body massage. Going further, to learn what's possible with massage outside pregnancy, you may want to look at *Sensual Massage for Couples* (Arcata Arts, 2002) Which details a full body massage that can last for an entire evening.

Massage for a Peaceful Pregnancy deals with a woman's body one part at a time. You will find strokes specifically designed for the hands, feet, legs, arms, head, back, and torso, but it's important to remember that most visible divisions of the body are only skin-deep. Simple toe massage might work up the sides of each toe a few times, corkscrewing, pulling, turning, and then, after a final squeeze, move on to the other foot. Nobody will fail to enjoy this brief sequence, but if you wish to view the toe as an organic part of the body, it's helpful to consider precisely which muscles allow it to move. Enter the complete toe massage, which begins up at the knee, where major toe muscles are anchored to bone. This kind of remote control of moving parts goes on all over the body: Fingers operate from the elbow, muscles used in lifting the arms run down the sides of the back, and the head is supported from between the shoulder blades. These are crucial relationships for a masseur who wishes to concentrate on a single part of the body.

Another crucial relationship, the one between a fetus and the surface of the mother's body, is apparent whenever you massage a pregnant woman. Their systems are in such close harmony that nearly everything is shared. Please the mother, and you benefit her child.

Although massage can be used instead of drugs to get rid of headaches, muscle cramps, and various

pains, it's much better to keep a woman relaxed so stress-related problems never have a chance to develop. Perhaps the best way to use this book is as a collection of pleasurable experiences that you can share with a pregnant woman. The stroke subheadings that follow offer an introduction to basic massage technique. Once the basic strokes have been learned, a masseur can adapt them to various parts of a pregnant woman's body. Examples of how to do this are offered throughout the book; as you work with a pregnant woman and learn to adapt massage to her changing needs, you will discover others.

All the strokes in the book were chosen because they feel remarkably good. Use them to please your partner throughout pregnancy and in the weeks following the birth of your new child.

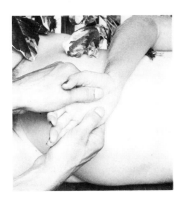

The immediate effects of massage are apparent on the skin. As surface circulation is stimulated a blush appears and surface tissues feel warm. With regular massage the skin becomes softer, more supple and begins to glow with a healthy radiance.

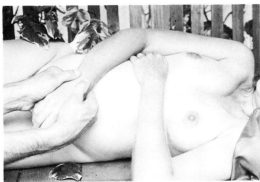

Some masseurs have a favorite "fallback" movement, something simple that's guaranteed to feel good no matter how much you've learned. When you're not sure what to do next rotate your forearm on the side of her leg or back and think it over.

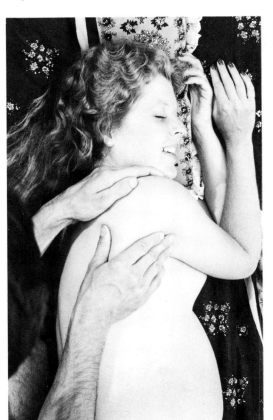

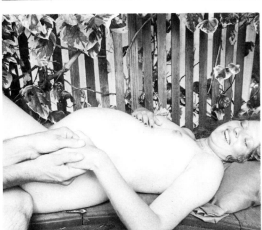

Friction

Friction is the fastest way to reach inside the body and make things happen. It should always be used at the beginning, rather than at the end, of a massage session because it leaves your partner stimulated. One variation of this movement, called spot friction, acts as a natural anesthetic and can be used independently of any other massage movement. The basic principle in every friction movement— that rubbing a sensitive spot produces relief—is understood instinctively by all mammals. That's hardly surprising because friction can be learned quickly and works almost immediately. It's a good way to begin massage, particularly if you want to get right into stress reduction and pain control. There's no need to oil the body; in fact, most friction movements are more effective without oil. Like every other massage stroke, friction, no matter where you use it, works best when your partner's whole body is relaxed. Always have her lie down before you begin.

Most friction movements will include only a limited part of the body. You might want to massage across the base of the neck and shoulders to give

relief to tensed muscles at the end of a day. Begin with a few minutes of friction, and then go on to fingertip kneading (see page 37). Spot friction techniques can be used to focus the movement on a specific point, like the center of a sore hip joint or the side of a knee. Inside the body, friction stirs up acidic waste products like lactic acid, dead cells, and the by-products of recent inflammations. It may take the body days to metabolize accumulated lactic acid that causes muscle exhaustion, but just a few minutes of friction can hasten the process and bring profound

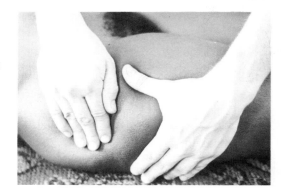

Deep Friction to the Hip:
The anchor hand—the hand that holds the body still—steadies the area just above the hip joint and presses down, gathering loose flesh, toward the friction hand. The fingers are held tightly together on the friction hand to increase contact. Pressure is concentrated on the whole surface of all four fingers while the hand is rotated on underlying tissue. Deep friction movements are ideal for stimulating the interior of large joints.

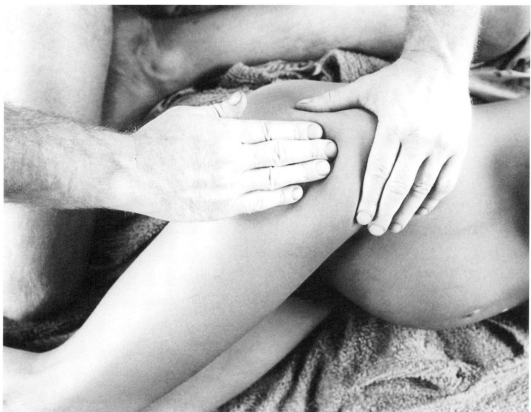

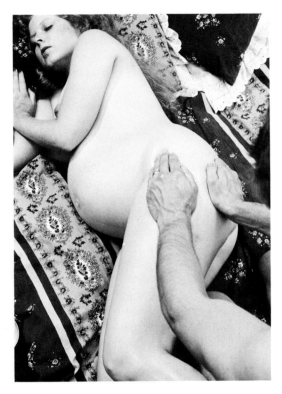

relief from fatigue (see "The Fluid Release Effect," page 44). Cell and tissue debris produce a dull, lethargic feeling that makes it difficult to find the energy for routine tasks. Here again, friction, followed by other massage strokes that stimulate circulation, can totally change your partner's mood. Every internal body change that takes place during pregnancy deposits chemical irritants in the surrounding tissues. This creates an extra burden that a pregnant woman can avoid if she is massaged regularly.

Friction strokes are particularly useful at the beginning of a massage if you want to leave your partner feeling more energetic when you're through.

The force used in doing friction is often much greater than is necessary. If redness and irritation be looked upon as a measure of the beneficial effects to friction upon the skin, then a coarse towel, a hair mitten, or a brush would answer for this purpose a great deal better than the hand alone.

Douglas Graham, MD

Friction

Variety	Technique	Effect
Surface Friction	Fingers apart, hand bends at the wrist; light pressure	Vibration on the skin surface; skin is "warmed"; circulation is improved
Medium Friction	Fingers together; anchor hand is sometimes necessary; wrist is rigid, whole arm turns; moderate pressure. Circle on top tissues, visible muscles, surface veins, nerves of the back	Stimulates nerves, improves circulation; stirs up tissue wastes
Deep Friction	Same as medium friction; anchor hand must be used; be sure you have good leverage; fatigue can be a problem; press down into the surface flesh. Circle near internal organs	Boosts arterial circulation; speeds lymphatic circulation; reaches blood vessels inside bones
Spot Friction	Focuses on one area; pressures will vary depending on the part of the body you're massaging; anchor hand continually picks up the same fold of flesh	A natural anesthetic

Percussion

Tapping on your partner's body produces a very pleasant vibration that will carry right through the whole torso or reach deep inside a limb. People who are afraid of massage find it easier to surrender and relax when a session begins with penetrating waves of pleasure. The sensation is so enjoyable that over the years a number of exotic gadgets have been developed in a desperate attempt to amplify the effects of "ordinary" massage. "Percussion Massage Devices of the Nineteenth and Twentieth Centuries," says the legend on an imaginary museum exhibit, and peering into a glassed box we find: tiny whips with india rubber balls on the tips; rubber handled wooden paddles that look suspiciously like Ping-Pong rackets; thimblelike finger caps with nasty little ball-points; overdecorated wooden talons which are permanently spread, like the claws of a blue-green lobster; and, from the South Pacific, palm fronds covered with tufts of matted animal hair. Swedish nudists experimented with lumpy strands of seaweed; which sounds like fun but could get sloppy. Farther to the south, a group of determined German scientists constructed

giant massage machines (some of them steam-powered and devilishly loud), in which huge iron gears spun a variety of lumpy wooden wheels, fluttering straps, brushes, gloves, and sponges against somebody's back. Happily no percussion device, from seaweed to steam engines, works nearly as well as human hands.

Many people are afraid to try percussion because the rapid "blows" look as though they could be painful. Actually percussion strokes are not blows at all; they are a kind of light tapping—a gentle rain, not a thunderstorm. As you learn the various movements, begin with very light tapping, and if your partner requests more pressure, gradually build up the intensity. The most important question is just how much pressure should be used during percussion movements. The only way to find out is to listen carefully to feedback from your partner while you're learning. Most women will ask for extra pressure, on the back and legs where thick muscle groups can absorb more vibration. Watch your hands when you do percussion, and be sure not to leave any kind of mark on your partner's skin. Red

Light Muscle Pounding:
The contact hand (his right) is fitted to the contour of the back and absorbs blows from the percussion hand. All percussion strokes must be cushioned so they do not become painful. To cushion further the force of light muscle pounding, the percussion hand bends at the wrist just before each "blow." The contact hand moves up and down the back and legs as this stroke continues. Light muscle pounding is particularly effective on the long muscles that run parallel to the spine and on the backs of the legs.

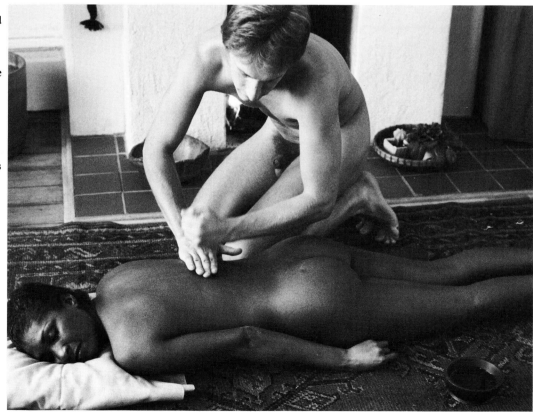

marks can become bruises the next day—a sad reminder of your attempts to relax and please her. Women will usually select a comfortable percussion level far below anything that could cause bruising.

The real purpose of every percussion movement is to create a cascading vibration that moves up and down the limbs and back. Most percussion strokes will work best on the back and on the backs of the legs. Stay away from exposed arteries (see illustration, page 100), the eyes, and bony parts of the body. Percussion strokes, combined with friction and kneading, are also wonderfully effective in relieving stress around a woman's shoulders and at the base of her neck. *Don't be afraid to go slowly; correct technique plus an even rhythm is more important than speed.*

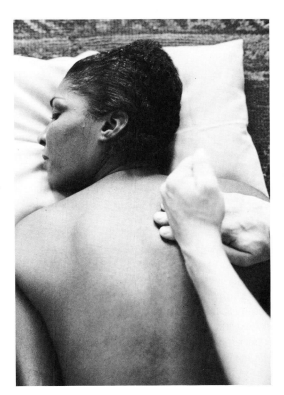

Vibrations of a certain strength and frequency given on a motor nerve set the corresponding muscles in action, and can produce an effect which is many hundred times greater than the force of the stimulus.

By pressure on the phrenic nerve where it can be reached in the neck it is possible to stop cramp in the diaphragm; by pressure on the spinal accessory nerve, cramp in that region, and the heart beat may be slowed by pressure on the vagus. (see p. 111)

Dr. Emil A.G. Kleen

Percussion

Variety	Technique	Effect
Hacking	Three middle fingers held together, lower finger hangs down to absorb the blow	Vibration just beneath the skin surface, very effective on the long muscles that run parallel to the spine
Tapping	Four fingertips of each hand contact a specific muscle group	Vibration to skin, top muscles, and nerves
Cupping	Hands curled with thumb pressed against forefinger, fingers held tightly together	Widespread vibration to all top tissues: flesh rises slightly as hands are lifted and "vacuum" effect is broken; good for side tissues of the back, buttocks, and backs of thigh
Thumping	One hand flat on the back, fingers together; the other hand strikes the center of the fingers with a closed fist; fist hand should bend at the wrist	Deep penetration to inner tissues; stimulates arterial circulation as well as the heart and lungs

Kneading

Kneading is the single most important movement in massage. It's effective on nearly every surface of the body and has a hypnotic rhythm that people find irresistible. Kneading "travels" very well from one part of the body to another; you can knead down the side of your partner's back and onto a leg or, if you prefer, turn at the hip and knead across to the other side of the back. Even the most delicate kneading strokes on the side of the face or around the eyes will reach underlying tissues and squeeze them several ways. This squeezing effect is an important part of the fluid release process, during which oxygen and blood-soluble nutrients are pumped into the tissues while acidic wastes are removed.

A thoroughly kneaded part of the body feels light and invigorated as though it had been rested for hours. Apart from the important physiological changes that take place during kneading, the stroke is immensely relaxing. Normally, during a full body massage, you might knead around the base of the back three times. But if you concentrate and repeat the kneading sequence an additional 100 times, the whole lower part of the body becomes transformed.

People who experience this for the first time are often surprised to learn that repetition of a single stroke can generate such a profound change.

Often when massage is mentioned in literature the specific reference is to kneading. Charlatans who use massage to promote themselves as magicians rely on ordinary kneading strokes to demonstrate their powers. Kneading is mentioned in Homeric literature, in the Bible, and in Oriental books that were probably written before the Bible. More than anything else, good kneading technique will make you a masseur and give you something to turn to everywhere on the body.

Full Hand Kneading the Thigh: The key to effective kneading is correct use of the thumbs. The hands move in rhythmic circles while the thumbs open and close. Each time a thumb opens, the opposing hand picks up a fold of flesh between the thumb and four fingers. On fleshy parts of the body, like the thigh, it's easy to pick up an ample fold of flesh whenever the thumbs close. Simply opening and closing the thumb preserves the kneading effect on bony areas, like the shoulder tops and ribs, where there isn't enough extra flesh to lift. Add oil to lubricate her skin and make kneading smooth and fluid.

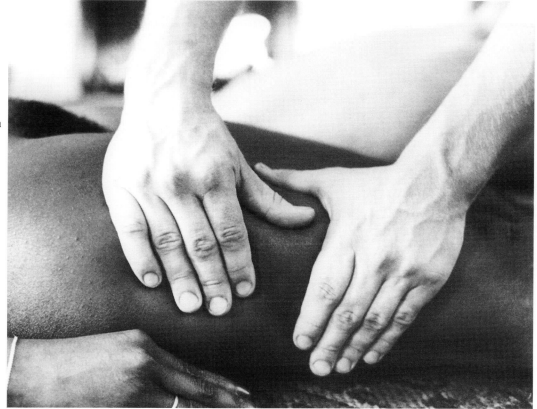

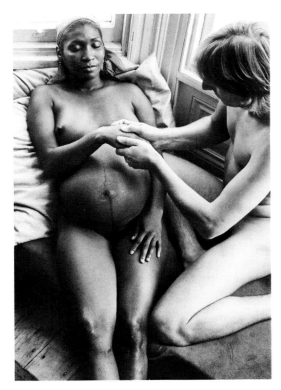
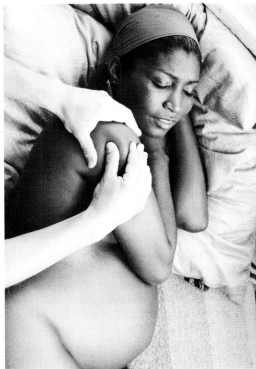

Deep kneading movements that reach interior muscles are particularly welcome after exercise or exertion. As acidic irritants are squeezed out of the tissues, soreness and stiffness disappear.

Kneading

Variety	Technique	Effect
Full-Hand Kneading	The whole surface of the hand, from the base of the palm to the tips of the fingers, is used; hands rotate in opposing circles	Tones muscles; promotes the fluid release effect; increases venous circulation; aids digestive process (over the abdomen)
Fingertip Kneading	Contact varies from fingertips only to first two digits of fingers; hands rotate in opposing cirles; thumb of each hand picks up some flesh every time a circle is made	Tones subcutaneous muscles; revitalizes skin
Closed-Hand Kneading	One hand moves exactly the same way as in full-hand kneading, while the other hand circles on the flat second knuckle	Deeper penetration than full-hand kneading; helps control localized pain; promotes arterial circulation; very effective on thickly muscled parts of the back and thighs

Stroking

Stroking will accelerate blood circulation almost anywhere in the body. Since a sense of well-being is closely tied to good blood circulation, it's usually the first major body change masseurs work to create. To understand just how much ordinary stroking movements can benefit your partner, it's useful to view the whole body as a river. When the flow is unimpeded, the water is clear, but as obstructions appear you begin to notice impurities. Stimulating circulation brings extra oxygen and blood-soluble nutrients to the tissues of the body. In just a few minutes you can triple the oxygen supply to a set of muscles while acidic wastes that cause irritation and fatigue are squeezed out and metabolized.

Every circulation movement is designed to aid the work of the heart as it pumps blood through the body. Strokes press in *toward* the heart with the full flat surface of your hands emptying underlying veins. Diminished pressure in the veins produces a temporary vacuum, and blood is immediately sucked in from nearby arteries with great force. During the stroking movement your hands and your partner's heart are working together to press

new blood into the veins and surrounding tissues. The first time that happens to her, your partner will discover a very pleasant body change that is unique to the massage experience: Blood will suddenly move more quickly through her body while the heart does *less* work.

The same stroking movements that work on blood vessels will also stimulate circulation in the lymphatic system, which has no heart and must depend entirely on body movement for the transfer of internal fluids. If your partner's pregnancy is so fatiguing that exercise has been completely abandoned, toxic fluids are likely to have stagnated throughout the lymphatic system. Stroking movements will flush out the whole system and leave her feeling refreshed.

Stroking may also be used to boost circulation to a specific part of the body and has a number of interesting therapeutic possibilities. You will notice a definite reduction in the swelling around a sprained ankle after a few minutes of friction and fingertip kneading followed by a stroking movement away from the sprain. In the later stages of pregnancy

Full-Hand Stroking the Torso: As the stroke travels from neck to hips, the hands adjust in order to mold themselves to your partner's torso. When her torso begins to change shape, you should maintain full contact from the fingertips to the bases of your palms. The hands begin in the center of the torso facing in opposite directions. Stroke across her torso until the fingertips of one hand and the wrist of the other touch the massage surface. Your thumbs brush lightly as the hands cross the center of her torso. Then reverse directions, and stroke to the other side of your partner's body. During pregnancy this stroke requires a light positive touch and plenty of oil.

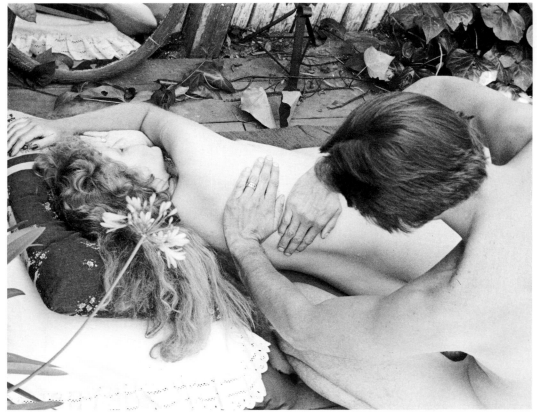

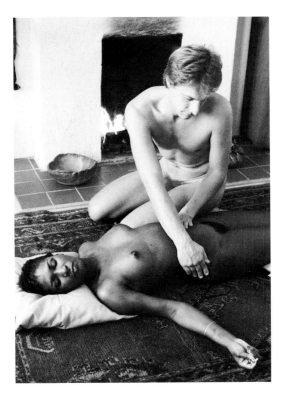

pressure from the expanded uterus on arteries to the legs can grow to the point where circulation below the waist becomes sluggish. Stroking movements on the feet and lower legs will leave these areas feeling rejuvenated. Generally this is the movement to use on any part of the body that feels sluggish and heavy.

Stroking movements can serve as a satisfying conclusion to the fluid release sequence (see page 44) or as a good introduction to massage. No movement is easier to learn. Rest assured, the first time you try stroking on a pregnant woman's arms and legs she will enjoy herself.

If you're concentrating on circulation instead of general massage straight line stroking movements should increase in velocity as they get further from the heart. Maintain a rate of ninety to one hundred eighty strokes per minute on the hands and feet.

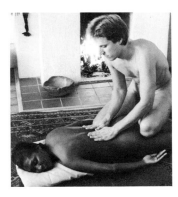

A common mistake: To gain a temporary advantage in leverage this masseur has placed himself in a position where repetition of the stroke will become difficult. Get comfortable at the beginning of a stroke and you won't have to interrupt your partner's massage.

Stroking

Variety	Technique	Effect
Full-Hand Stroking	Usually used on limbs or torso; the whole surface of the hand, from the base of the palm to the fingertips, makes contact; on thin parts of the limbs the hands should assume a cupped shape to maintain full contact; hands push in opposite directions	Promotes blood and lymph circulation; tones blood vessels; relieves sluggishness and fatigue
One-Hand Stroking	Identical to full-hand stroking, but the hands move up limbs one at a time; helpful when extra pressure or speed is desired	Promotes blood and lymph circulation; tones blood vessels; relieves sluggishness and fatigue; good for fast stroking away from sprains

Passive Exercise

Passive exercise, a technique masseurs share with physical therapists, allows you to move parts of a woman's body without asking her to use any muscle power. Physical therapists working on disabled patients use passive exercises to restore mobility to muscles that have been out of use because of sickness or injury. Moving any part of an invalid's body will stimulate and strengthen the heart. But if you want to build muscles, merely rotating or pulling a leg cannot compare to actually walking or running on it.

To a masseur, the real value in passive exercise is the gratifying way it can be used to stretch the internal structures of joints throughout the body. A supple joint is largely dependent on the flexibility of internal ligaments and tendons. Stiff joints can remain tight right through a rigorous exercise program, and sadly they often do. We have all seen the marathoner who continues for hours with rigid, jerky upper body movements. The legs are moving smoothly, but are the shoulders? A slight change in the way the joints work makes every motion more fluid and natural.

Like most moving parts in any complicated machine, human joints require internal lubrication. It's supplied by a creamy substance, called synovial fluid, which is stored in a series of membranes around every joint. Passive exercises will stimulate the production of this vital material and effectively squirt it onto the joint's surfaces. But manipulating the joint does much more than "oil" the contact surfaces. It also stretches internal ligaments that connect the joint to surrounding bones and puts tension on the tendons that connect muscles to the joint.

Every major joint near the center of the body changes position as the fetus develops. Inside each joint ligaments and tendons will stretch to accommodate the growing womb, but if a woman's body is not well conditioned, the process can be painful and very tedious. Passive exercises, used regularly over the course of a pregnancy, will keep the joints supple and allow internal ligaments and tendons to stretch gracefully as your child grows.

The Full Body Lift:
The best way to lift is from a simple tripod position with one knee down and one foot flat. This allows you to balance yourself easily and lift your partner to a comfortable position. The hands are clasped, fingers intertwined, beneath the small of her back. As you lift, your partner's head and shoulders will fall back gracefully. Raising and lowering her at the same speed allow her to relax each time the stroke is repeated. Lift to a point that's comfortable for both of you. As the back is lifted, intervertebral ligaments of the lower spine and nearby tendons are gently stretched.

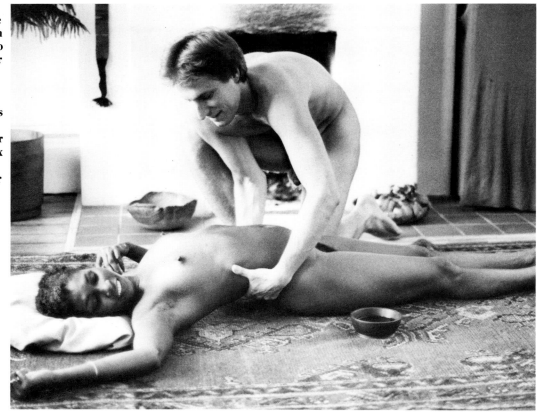

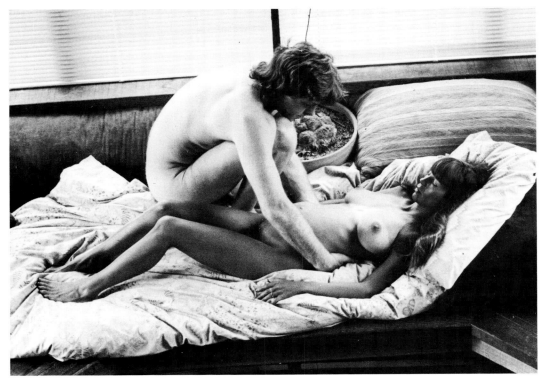

Passive exercises are used to move sections of a woman's body while she remains completely relaxed. You explore the range of movement that's available to a joint while your partner does nothing at all. After the birth, passive exercises become resistive exercises as the two of you work together to recondition the new mother's body.

Passive Exercise

Variety	Technique	Effect
Rotation	Lift (leg, arm, finger, toe, hand, or foot), and rotate at joint just inside the point where resistance is felt	Lubricates the joint
Rotate and Pull	Find convenient natural "handle" to grasp and pull back as you rotate; the legs and feet usually accept lots of pressure while you pull back	Lubricates the joint and stretches internal ligaments and tendons; pulling the top and bottom of the foot will affect joints at the hip, knee, and ankle
Lift and Shake	Give good support to the legs, arms, and around the small of the back when you lift; gentle, rhythmic shaking is best	Lubricates the joint; improves internal circulation

Sensation Transfers

Each stroke you do during a massage adds to a reservoir of feelings that can eventually spread throughout the whole body. Massage a leg, and you fill it with the most delicious sensations. Your partner's mind will focus on that leg and the feeling you've just created. If you suddenly begin massaging the other leg (or an arm), the transition can be too quick and a bit confusing. Sensation transfers allow your partner to experience a delicate feeling that will move slowly off the part of the body you've just massaged and finally come to rest on the next place where you intend to work.

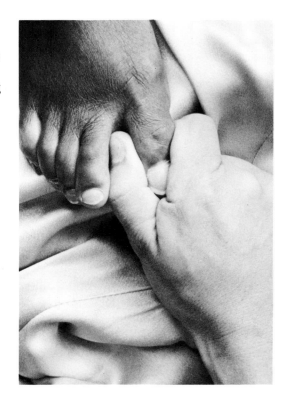

Even if many sensations were cut off, if you were surrounded by complete darkness and silence, if there were nothing to smell or taste, if you were floating weightless in space and could feel nothing, there would still be sensations arising from your own muscles and joints to tell you the relative position of your limbs and torso.

Isaac Asimov

Sensation Transfers

Variety	Technique	Effect
Body Brushing	With fingertips of both hands wide open, sweep down the body usually away from the heart	Soothes the nerves; "connects" one part of the body to another as you massage
Brushing with the Hair	Bend your head, and let your hair run across the part of the body just massaged	Unique and delightful sensation; "connects" one part of the body to another as you massage
Blowing	Take a deep breath, and blow lightly down the length of the limb you've just massaged	Most delicate sensation transfer

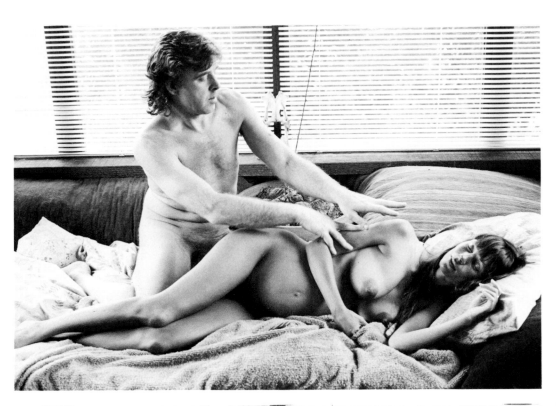

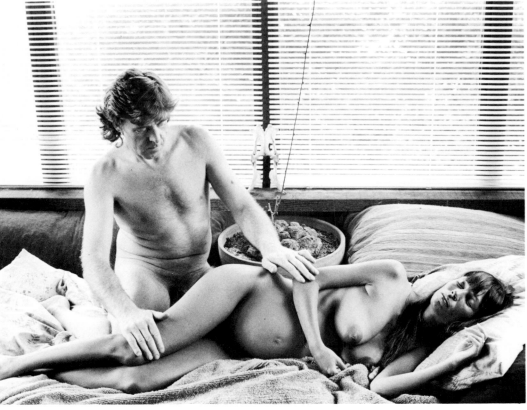

Transferring Sensation from the Arms to the Legs:
Fingers are held in an open, relaxed position as the hands brush down your partner's arm one after another. Brushing speed varies and grows progressively lighter. Eventually only the fingertips of one hand remain in contact with your partner's arm. Your free hand initiates contact with the leg the moment arm contact is broken.

43

The Fluid Release Effect

Just before the turn of the century, when doctors still found time to massage a patient, French medical researchers demonstrated how effective different movements were in promoting good health. Almost every body process was examined before and after massage in order to determine exactly what benefits could be derived from the repetition of various movements. When stroking began, the heart rate and blood pressure immediately decreased.

The researchers observed how stagnant lymph flowed abundantly the moment an area was massaged and noted an increased sodium chloride level in sweat and tears after a session. Their most important discovery for pregnant women, however, is the way certain massage movements can be used to eliminate tension-causing chemicals that collect in the body's tissues. This is the fluid release effect, a feature that can enhance almost any massage, particularly if a woman is suffering from fatigue or stress. Masseurs view stress as a physical problem and deal with it by making gentle changes occur inside a woman's body.

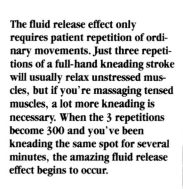

The fluid release effect only requires patient repetition of ordinary movements. Just three repetitions of a full-hand kneading stroke will usually relax unstressed muscles, but if you're massaging tensed muscles, a lot more kneading is necessary. When the 3 repetitions become 300 and you've been kneading the same spot for several minutes, the amazing fluid release effect begins to occur.

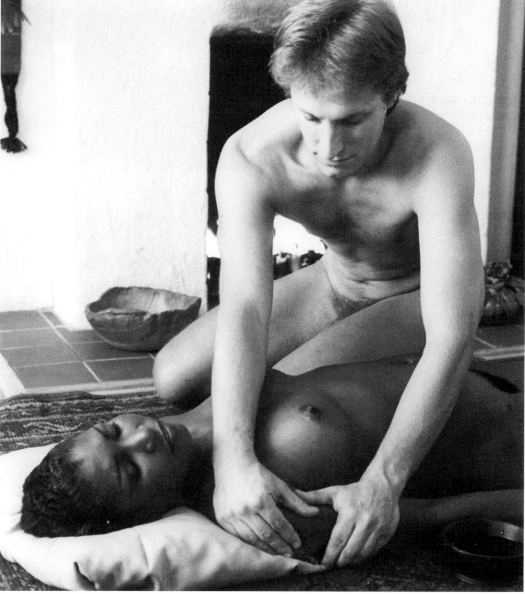

Every muscle fiber, skin cell, and nerve ending requires nutrition as well as oxygen in order to function. Soluble nutrients and oxygen are carried by the blood to all parts of the body. They combine and combust wherever energy is needed. Immediately after combustion, various gases, toxins, and wastes are produced; these must then be expelled from the tissues (and later from the body) via the complex venous and lymphatic systems. Combustion and waste elimination each depend on a vigorously healthy circulatory system. Unfortunately stress causes the vascular system to contract while all bodily secretions decrease. The familiar pale, waxy complexion that afflicts habitually tense people indicates that vascular circulation has become sluggish. When this happens, combustion is impeded and acidic wastes begin to accumulate in the tissues. This leaves a woman feeling irritable, fatigued and helpless because nothing she does seems to improve her condition.

Exercise will temporarily boost combustion rates, only to leave the muscles filled with a new waste, called lactic acid, which causes the same kind of pain and cramping athletes come to dread. Whether a woman exercises or not, fluid release massage strokes will pump oxygen and nutrients into the tissues while irritating wastes are removed. She will rise from the massage surface feeling refreshed and invigorated because you have made her body work more efficiently.

After five minutes of full-hand kneading, combustion and waste elimination are dramatically boosted. Oxygen levels in the affected tissues rise by 15 percent, while the number of red and white corpuscles increase by 55 and 85 percent respectively. The recovery rate of exhausted muscles is significantly shorter, and women often report that physical work is easier after a few minutes of massage than after an hour of bed rest.

During a fluid release sequence toxins and acidic irritants that can take days to seep through the intricate lymphatic system are pressed out as the muscles are continually squeezed like a sponge. Urinalysis reveals that the production of gastric juice, saliva, and urea is stimulated during massage, while nitrogen, sugar, and inorganic phosphorus excretion increases. Many of these benefits were observed one full week after a single massage session during which fluid release techniques were used!

After five minutes of Fluid Release Massage . . .

System	Effect	Result
Vascular	Blood supply to the massage site is tripled.	Blood vessels are "toned," the heart rate slows, the pulse drops, venous return valves are exercised, blood pressure is lowered.
Blood	The oxygen content of the tissues is boosted 10 or 15%. Red and white blood cell counts are increased by more than 50%.	Combustion of stored energy and fats is more efficient. Pain levels are reduced.
Nervous	Nerve endings are cleared of microscopic debris. Direct pressure on nerves is relieved as nearby muscles relax.	Tension levels are reduced. Muscles around the spine relax. Internal organs work more efficiently. Clear thinking.
Skin	Dead brittle skin is removed, the sebaceous secretion is stimulated on the scalp.	The skin takes on a healthy glow, superficial facial wrinkles begin to disappear, the hair looks glossy and moisturized.
Muscular	Lactic acid and other irritating wastes are squeezed out. Internal blood supply triples.	Muscle recovery rates after exercise are more than doubled, movement becomes light and effortless, an energized feeling pervades the muscles and surrounding tissues.

Improvisation and Repetition

Once mastered, the more than 140 movements involved in a full body massage provide the basis for all kinds of experimentation. A kneading movement on the side of the back that usually runs from the armpit to the pelvic bone can just as easily extend from the shoulder to the knee. Friction movements that concentrate on the back of the knee, where an intricate web of ligaments and muscles intertwine, can move down onto the larger calf muscles. Even the most subtle facial movements that create just a single sensation across the eyelids can be blended with temple stroking so that one sensation becomes two.

A full body massage that would usually last an hour and a half can go on to include dozens of new movements that have no name and have never been described. People who get massaged regularly learn to cherish the variety that comes with sensitive improvisation. In fact this enthusiasm can be so contagious that a new masseur may get carried away and begin drifting across the body deliriously improvising strange movements. Unfortunately, since your instrument is the human body, not a

piano, you just can't get away with this. Massaging half a muscle group on the back of the neck and then dancing over to tickle an ear may look smashing, but it will leave your partner unsatisfied.

Once you understand how important, say, fluid release massage is to a pregnant woman, it's easy to remain on the shoulders when you could be darting around the back and legs. When in doubt, be generous and continue with a stroke. If repeating a single kneading movement 300 times seems dull, remember that your partner is definitely not getting bored. Let the feeling go on. It's what *she* feels and what's going on inside that matter.

An extra twenty kneading strokes to a tensed arm and shoulder can put an insomniac to sleep. If your partner falls asleep while you're massaging it's a sign that what you were doing is working. More massage while she's asleep will continue to benefit her body.

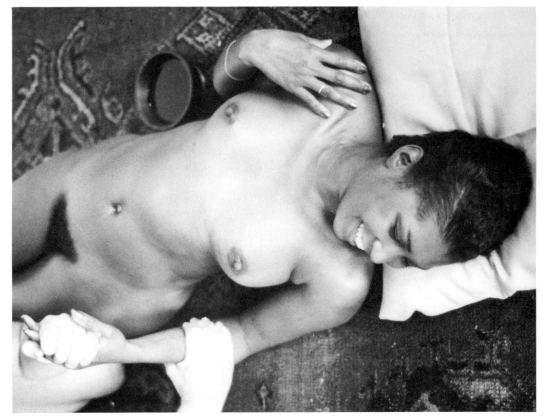

EARLY
PREGNANCY

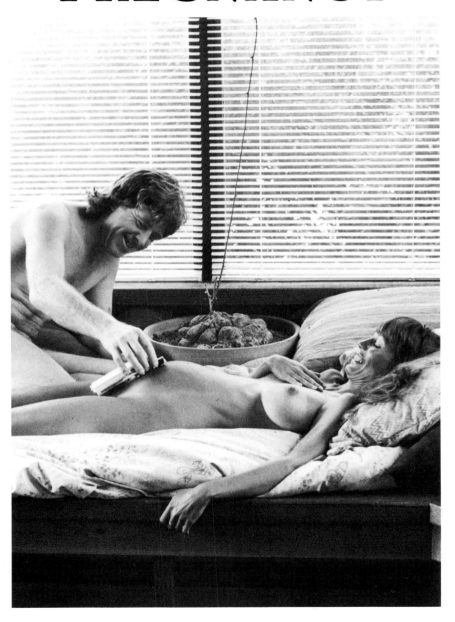

The Benefits of a First Massage During Pregnancy

One of the initial things you accomplish in a first massage during pregnancy is to awaken the skin and introduce your partner to a new range of pleasant feelings. Even though the skin is the body's largest organ, most people pay very little attention to the messages they receive from it. The skin will let you know if you're too hot or too cold, and of course, it registers pain. These are some of life's most familiar sensations, so regular and predictable that people take little notice. Most waking hours the skin is wrapped in neutral feeling fabrics that effectively attenuate all sensory messages. For many people a normal body is one that feels nothing, and almost any kind of sensation indicates a problem. A pregnant woman whose body is changing daily will not be well served by this kind of conditioning. When you awaken her body with massage, she learns that new sensations can be a pleasant surprise, not merely cause for alarm.

It's important to go slowly during a first massage to heighten a pregnant woman's basic sensory awareness. Usually, when adults choose to feel an object, they will explore it with the palm side of the hand. That part of the body contains less than one percent of the skin's surface. A slow first massage allows a woman to feel with the "unused" 99 percent of her body. As you move from head to toe, a woman will discover hundreds of new sensations.

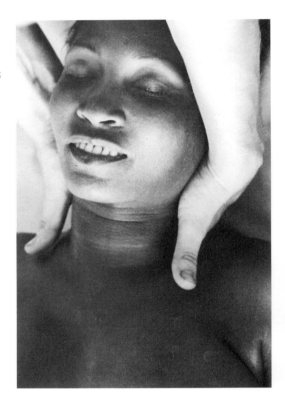

There's always one special point during a first massage, perhaps when a single toe rises and begins to turn independently of the others, when a woman discovers that her whole body is a friendly place where pleasurable things can happen. As her masseur you become part of this process, making your point physically, not just intellectually. She can feel that you accept her body as it grows and changes.

The sense organs are primed to note changes rather than absolute or static conditions. Indeed, the body tends to adapt to reasonable environmental conditions. We "tune out" until something new or different occurs.

Lennart Nilsson

Basic Massage for Early Pregnancy

Movement	Uses
Full-Hand Friction	Interior muscles and organs
Stroking	Large, flat areas, like the torso and back
Circulation (a stroking variation)	The limbs and back
Full-Hand Kneading	Larger, fleshy areas, like the thighs, calves, and sides of the spine
Fingertip Kneading	Small, uneven bony areas, like the hands and feet; also used on the arms
Percussion	The lungs and the backs of the legs
Passive Exercise	The lower back and limbs

Morning Sickness and Massage

In the first months of pregnancy you can use massage to deal with the unpredictable effects of morning sickness. A woman's body changes so rapidly that it's often difficult to pinpoint the exact cause of a problem. Is an unexpected spate of headaches caused by the normal increase in blood volume and heart rate temporarily straining the cerebral blood vessels or by purely emotional tension, causing spasm of the sternocleidomastoid muscles of the neck? Is dizziness caused by anemia, which may call for dietary supplements, or by stress-induced hyperventilation? Are leg cramps related to too much calcium in the diet or to poor circulation and overstrained muscles? Massage is a very powerful tool and will provide drugless solutions to many of the problems that pregnant women might face. However, if a problem is serious enough to cause real discomfort, it's probably a good idea to see a doctor. The stakes are very high during pregnancy, and a masseur should always pay close attention to a physician's advice. Once you're certain that, say, fatigue is not related to malnutrition, you can begin clearing the lymphatic system and refreshing the whole body.

At any stage in a pregnancy there are persistent problems that may be annoying but not serious enough for a visit to the doctor. Right at the top of that list is morning sickness, the bane of many early pregnancies. Can massage help? If a woman is reacting to increased progesterone and hCG levels in her blood, the problem is hormonal, and she won't be helped by massage, medicine, or religion. Just leave her alone, and try to keep everything warm and quiet. Like all of life's problems, hormonally induced morning sickness will pass.

Nausea is the most difficult aspect of morning sickness for a masseur to deal with because while it's going on, physical contact is usually not desirable. Afterward, when the distressing symptoms have subsided, you can begin to experiment with stress reduction techniques in the hope that the cause of her suffering is not purely hormonal. Then massage will bring blessed relief without requiring a woman to resort to Benedictine or megavitamin therapy. The area on the mid-spine where direct nerve connections to the digestive organs are found (see illustration, page 111) is certainly worth a few extra minutes of friction and fingertip kneading whenever you massage her. Work on nausea in the evening, when the whole body is more likely to be settled.

Fortunately most other causes of morning sickness will respond much more favorably to massage. Intense nervousness can bring on most morning sickness symptoms in a few minutes, and masseurs have seen them disappear just as quickly. A hundred years ago the term "neurasthenia" was used to describe a general irritability that could lead to a host of unhappy afflictions. Today the concept is considered too broad to be useful, but the condition still exists and is particularly troublesome during pregnancy. Recently psychologists have modernized the whole notion and managed to find, in the balmy days of early pregnancy, enough angst, despair, and ambivalence to motivate Ph.D. candidates for the next few decades. The research on this phenomenon is already much more frightening than the problem itself, and a woman who analyzes her "emotional ambivalence" or struggles to understand a "rejection conflict" will soon know, intimately, the kind of stress that leads to morning sickness. Once the nausea has subsided, you can use basic massage sequences to soothe the nerves and bring drugless relief.

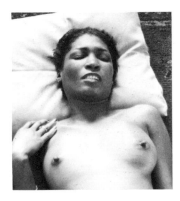

Morning sickness usually means suffering at the beginning of the day. Don't let occasional headaches and nausea define a woman's pregnancy. You can add pleasure to her life later in the same day with massage.

3

Full-Hand Friction for the Backs of the Legs and the Back

Friction strokes are an easy way to begin massaging without oil (although you can also use them after you've oiled), particularly if your partner has been suffering from muscular pain or fatigue. A deep, penetrating full-hand friction stroke will bring immediate relief, after which you can oil the body and continue with general massage.

Fast friction tends to anesthetize local nerves while slow friction stimulates them. If you decide on fast friction, select a speed that you can maintain comfortably. Intermittent bursts of speed will confuse your partner and limit your endurance. Press down hard enough so that your hands do not move across your partner's skin. During friction, you can actually feel internal muscles and organs beneath the skin; rotate on *them*. Most friction movements are easier to focus if you stabilize a part of the body with one hand and apply friction with the other.

The hand that holds the body still, called the *anchor hand,* must gather up a fold of flesh between the thumb and forefinger and press in toward the area where you want to apply friction. This creates a loose skin effect that allows the surface tissues to move as you penetrate deep within you partner's body. Your friction stroke can travel up and down the back and thigh, but remember not to break contact when your hands move.

If you're right-handed (left-handed people should reverse this technique), anchor your left hand against the back of your partner's thigh, and press in toward the first spot where you want to do some friction. Once you've gathered a small fold of flesh, press down immediately in front of it with your friction hand. Use as much of your hand as possible, and allow it to shape itself to the contour of your partner's thigh. Press down and rotate on the interior muscles. Massage in circles, concentrating on one spot for a while and then moving up and down the thigh until you've covered the whole area. Use supporting pillows and lots of pressure over the calf. Decrease your pressure over soft internal organs below the bottom ribs.

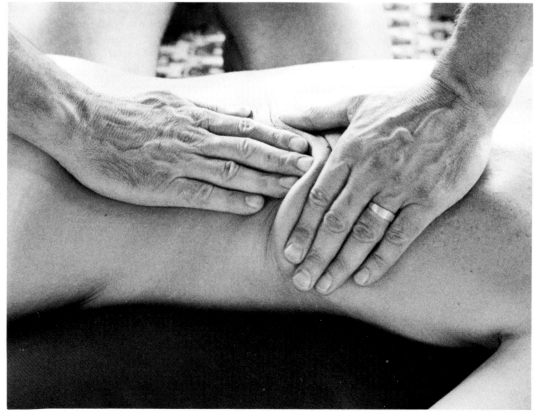

Full-Hand Stroking on the Back

Full-hand stroking covers the entire center of the back and can easily be modified for use on the arms and legs. It follows the whole length of the internal erector muscles that run parallel to the spine and hold it in place. This is where many of the cramps associated with serious back problems originate. Keeping these muscles supple in the early stages of pregnancy will allow them to adapt more easily to increased strains in the months to come, when most of the extra abdominal weight must be borne by muscles that tie into the lower back.

Even in the earliest stages of pregnancy it's a good idea to use plenty of extra padding beneath a woman's midsection before you massage her back. This is a good time to dig into your pillow collection once again or to bring out a few thick blankets. Once the extra padding has been covered with a sheet that feels comfortable to her, you're ready to oil your partner's back.

You can effectively massage the back from either side, but the very best position for center strokes like this one is simply to straddle your partner. That way you can reach all the way up the center of her back to the shoulders without favoring either side. When you need to rest, sitting back on your legs for a while won't put any extra pressure on your partner's abdomen. Straddling makes it easy for you to balance movements up the center center of her back and distribute pressures evenly with both hands.

Begin with both hands cupping your partner's shoulders, and pull one hand all the way down to her waist. Keep the entire surface of your hand, from the fingertips to the base of the palm, in contact with her back. Hold your fingers together as you pull the hand down, and allow your thumb to "ride" in the slight depression right next to her spine. By using the thumb as a guide, you can prevent the pressure part of the stroke from ever touching the spine. Direct pressure on the spine is risky; avoid it whenever you massage the back.

As soon as one hand reaches the waist, reverse direction, and begin the trip back up to the shoulders, following exactly the same path you used on the way down. As one hand begins to rise from the waist, the other hand should start down.

You can change this stroke to a very effective circulation movement for the whole back by simply moving up from the bottom of the back with both hands together. Your hands separate just below your partner's neck and turn outward across the shoulder tops. The return part of the stroke uses light pressure as you move down the sides of her body to the starting point at the bottom of the back. Go easy on the lowest part of her back below the rib cage.

The two hands pass each other, thumbs nearly touching, midway between the shoulders and waist. Each time you reach a shoulder be sure to bend your fingers around it. Small courtesies make the difference between a massage that's merely adequate and one that's unforgettable.

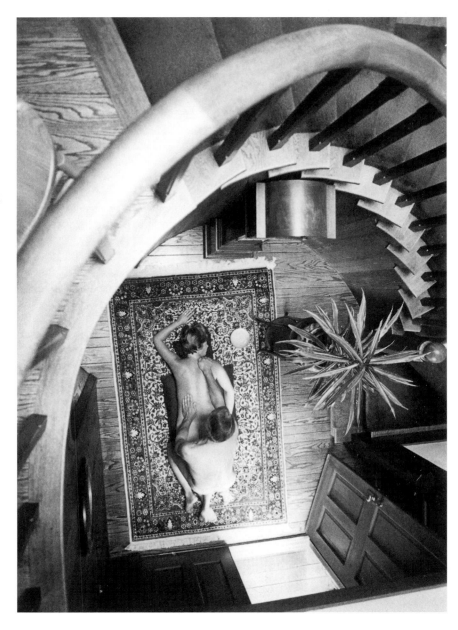

3

Keeping the Veins Healthy

The contracting hands of the [masseur] are, as it were, two more propelling hearts at the peripheral ends of the circulation cooperating with the one at the centre, and the analogy will not suffer if we bear in mind that the size of one's heart is about as large as the shut hand, and the number of intermittent squeezes of massage that act most favorably on vessels, muscles, and nerves are about seventy-two per minute, which is about the ordinary pulse rate. If this is not an art that does mend nature, what is?

Douglas Graham

Ordinary kneading, friction, and circulation movements will pump blood through every part of her legs without speeding up the heart. It takes only a few minutes to bring the venous blood supply up to *triple* the normal rate. No extra strain is put on the heart to achieve this.

In early pregnancy increased pressure on the veins, caused by a quickened heart rate and greater blood volume, can lead to a rash of annoying headaches (see page 70). Once you've massaged the head, neck, and shoulders to relieve the pain, it's a good idea to give some attention to the extremities. If the head was congested, you can be almost certain that venous circulation is impeded elsewhere—usually in the legs, hands, or feet.

Exercise is the traditional way of keeping the veins supple, but unfortunately a certain amount of inactivity is almost inevitable during pregnancy. Difficult days will come, and when they do, a woman may have to stay off her feet and take it easy for a while. Doing nothing while feeling slightly ill can be particularly frustrating for the active woman who is accustomed to feeling fit and ready to go. She must suddenly adapt to body changes which are difficult to predict and utterly beyond her control. An entire morning of dizziness and nausea doesn't put anyone in the mood for vigorous exercise, even though that might be just what's needed to prevent the unpleasantness from recurring.

Prolonged inactivity, in fact, generates a new set of problems for the pregnant woman: Muscle tone decreases, body weight increases, and circulation become sluggish. Without good circulation, digestion, respiration, resistance to disease, and virtually every other body process are degraded. The weakest systems are first to be affected, and a general feeling of weariness is likely to be followed by a specific ailment (like an infection) that stubbornly hangs on much longer than it should. Pregnant women are most vulnerable in the legs, where pressures from the growing womb on abdominal arteries can impede circulation in the lower body. If the cycle of illness and inactivity continues, a woman runs the risk of developing varicose veins, which is always a potential problem during pregnancy (particularly if other women in her family have been sufferers).

With a basic understanding of how the venous system works, you can use massage to keep the veins healthy throughout pregnancy. Veins are thicker and stronger than arteries and have twice

the capacity. Both advantages tend to compensate for decreased pressure in the venous system as blood returns to the heart from the ends of high-pressure arteries. The action of voluntary muscles pressing against the veins while performing ordinary tasks like walking further helps with the work. As blood is returned to the heart, valves within individual veins prevent it from backflowing and pooling in the legs. Problems usually begin when too much time is spent standing motionless, sitting, or resting and the beneficial effect of leg motion on circulation is lost. Eventually the veins begin to lose their tone, a valve fails, and they become dilated, as the swollen unsightly blue cords known as varicosities begin to appear.

During pregnancy varicose veins are more likely to occur in the left leg than in the right. The reason for this is not known, but it may be due to

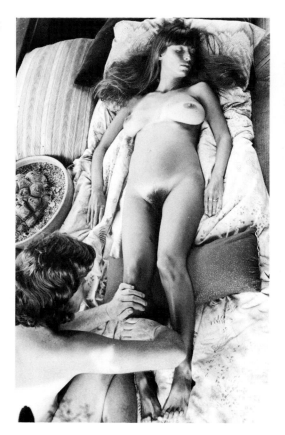

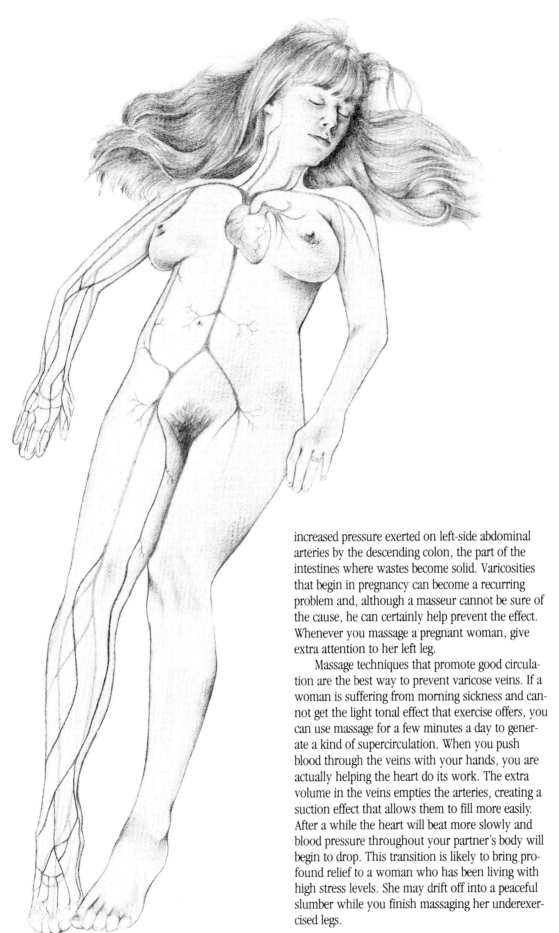

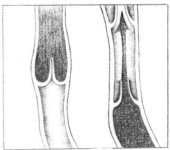

As blood from the capillary beds of the legs is returned to the heart against the flow of gravity it is prevented from backflowing by tiny valves that will only open towards the heart. Since the vein walls are not rigidly muscular like the sides of arteries these valves are crucial to an even distribution of blood throughout the legs. They appear irregularly along the main veins, usually at intersections between the deep and superficial blood vessels of the lower leg. Keep them in mind when you massage the leg and give extra attention to the area below the knee.

increased pressure exerted on left-side abdominal arteries by the descending colon, the part of the intestines where wastes become solid. Varicosities that begin in pregnancy can become a recurring problem and, although a masseur cannot be sure of the cause, he can certainly help prevent the effect. Whenever you massage a pregnant woman, give extra attention to her left leg.

Massage techniques that promote good circulation are the best way to prevent varicose veins. If a woman is suffering from morning sickness and cannot get the light tonal effect that exercise offers, you can use massage for a few minutes a day to generate a kind of supercirculation. When you push blood through the veins with your hands, you are actually helping the heart do its work. The extra volume in the veins empties the arteries, creating a suction effect that allows them to fill more easily. After a while the heart will beat more slowly and blood pressure throughout your partner's body will begin to drop. This transition is likely to bring profound relief to a woman who has been living with high stress levels. She may drift off into a peaceful slumber while you finish massaging her underexercised legs.

Hand-Over-Hand Circulation

This is the classic circulation stroke used in almost every massage to push blood back toward the heart. It's effective on both sides of each limb, on the feet, and, in an altered form, on the back and torso. Women love the way it feels and will not be disappointed if you continue for a long time. And why don't you? Circulation strokes increase the blood flow within local tissues while slowing down the heart. There is, quite simply, no way, outside of massage, for a human being to experience this. Make it last.

Wrap your hands around the bottom of your partner's leg or arm just above the foot or hand with the fingers pointing in opposite directions. When massaging the front of the left arm or leg, begin with your right hand on top. The starting position is reversed on the other limb and on the backs of the legs. (This stroke is not useful on the backs of the arms.) The correct starting position allows your hands to turn properly at the top of the limb. There your top hand should glide over the top of the shoulder or across the hip as both hands turn to descend down the sides. Keep your fingers

together throughout the stroke, and practice it until the whole thing runs smoothly and there is no obvious repositioning of your hands at any point.

Both sides of the lower arm can be effectively massaged with circulation strokes from the front of the body. (From the back, your partner's elbow will prevent you from using this stroke on the whole arm.) Turn her palm down to massage the back of the arm. With the palm up, her arm will bend away from the body at the elbow, revealing the "carrying angle," the position of the lower arm in relation to her torso. This exposes the soft, fleshy part of the forearm, where circulation strokes are particularly effective. Lift the arm with both hands when you turn it to give her an extra sense of security.

Remember to keep your hands locked together until they begin to separate at the top of the limb. To benefit the venous system, most of your pressure should be toward the heart. Light contact will do on the return stroke down the side of the limb.

A common circulation stroke mistake: The masseur began his partner's left arm with his left hand on top. If he wishes to turn gracefully at the top of the stroke, he will have to stop just below her armpit, omitting the entire shoulder.

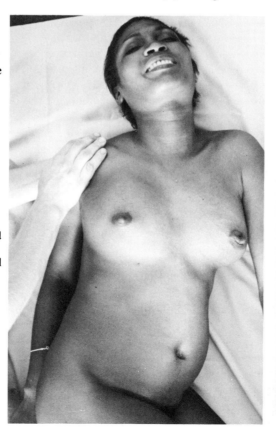

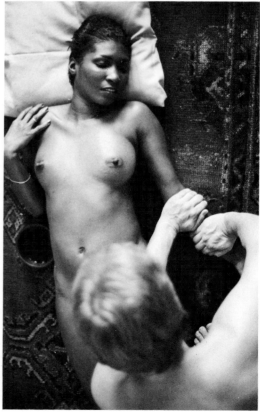

High-Pressure Circulation

Here is a circulation stroke that permits you to bear down and direct pressure onto the veins while you press forward toward the heart. It's an easy way to concentrate the circulation effect on a specific part of an arm or leg where your partner needs extra attention. This is the ideal way to begin massaging a cramped or cold limb. High-pressure circulation brings a sudden rush of warmth wherever it's used.

One hand presses toward the heart, and as it lifts to return to the starting position, the other hand moves forward. Move the starting position up and down a limb as you continue stroking. Whether you move up or down, your hands should always press toward the heart as they stroke. High-pressure circulation, repeated many times, is invigorating.

The area covered by your stroking can vary, depending on what you want to do. Just above the knee a series of short, rapid strokes will adequately focus the circulation effect. Strokes that are nearly half a leg long are useful if you want to move up and down the entire limb. On the foot you can push forward over a very small area, hardly more than a hand's width wide.

Extra speed doesn't necessarily mean more pressure. Try to keep your stroking even, and arrange your own body before starting this stroke to prevent early fatigue from stretching. You get good leverage on your partner's foot by positioning yourself just below it. If you're planning to stroke the entire leg, sit near the knee (as shown), where you can easily reach back to the foot, and from there press forward all the way up to her hip. The arm can be stroked from below or along the side.

There's plenty of repetitious contact in this stroke, and you should be prepared to add oil if her skin begins to dry out. The moment your hands begin to pull on her skin, it's time for more oil.

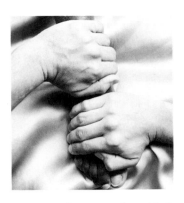

Keep your fingers together with the hands cupped enough to ensure a snug fit around every part of the foot or limb you're massaging. Stroking speed can vary according to what you can manage comfortably and what your partner enjoys, but save your very fastest strokes for the feet, where venous circulation tends to be sluggish. Veins there are very close to the surface and easily constricted by modern shoes.

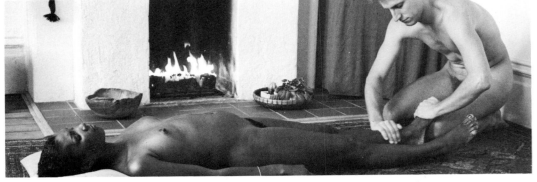

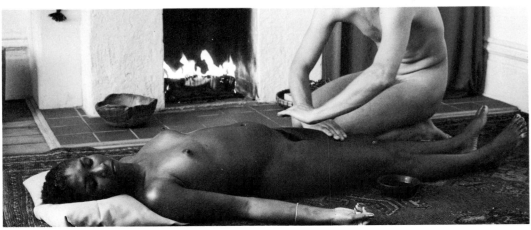

Understanding Cramps

Muscles move the body by contracting, and a cramp occurs when a contracted muscle "freezes" and cannot return to a relaxed state. Cramps are largely a result of poor circulation not just to the affected muscle but to a whole portion of the body. They occur most frequently in the extremities, where a sudden chill can bring on a cramp in less than a minute. When circulatory patterns begin to change in early pregnancy, sudden cramps will often strike odd parts of the body and badly frighten a woman. They can continue into late pregnancy, when the weight of the uterus puts pressure on arteries to the legs. Massage can make a major difference in nearly every cramp, particularly when the problem seems to occur in the same place. You can end a cramp soon after it begins and prevent it from ever returning. In both cases your main objective is to relax and oxygenate interior tissues around the cramped area.

Cramps can precipitate a variety of other morning sickness problems if they strike near dawn, suddenly awakening a woman from sleep. This can become a recurring problem and is particularly troublesome in the winter months, when the lower legs tend to become chilled at night. The attack can come without any warning and, if nothing is done to relieve the pain, will usually last long enough to frighten a pregnant woman. Typically the cramped part of the body will bend into an exaggerated curve. The arch of the foot becomes terribly severe, a leg is twisted oddly at the knee, or the whole body is bent over at the waist. In the dead of night, when there are few distractions, pain always seems more intense.

In each case the first step in relieving a cramp is to stretch out the afflicted part of the body until it reaches the normally relaxed position. Press the cramped area back into a normal position. Once you've done that, you can begin pumping oxygen into the cramped muscles with circulation, kneading, and friction strokes. Cramps are frightening but not that serious. Remaining calm while you relax a strained muscle will aid in solving the problem and allow a woman to trust you the next time you propose using massage to help her through a difficult period.

Adults will usually close their eyes the moment massage begins. Doing so immediately amplifies the tactile sense and brings on deep relaxation. When massaging a cramp, however, you may have to remind your partner to close her eyes. The darkness helps her let go and relax while you work on the painful area.

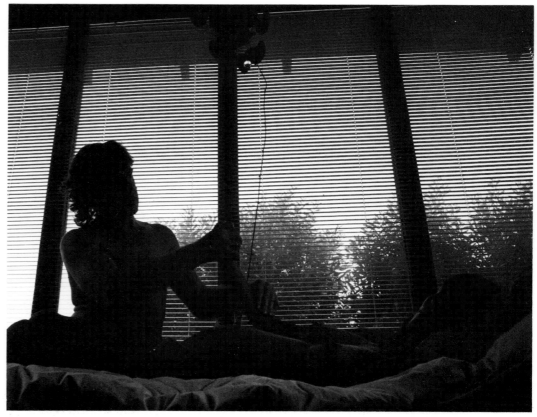

Full-Hand Kneading

Layers of thick muscles and soft, fleshy tissues respond well to kneading. The backs of the legs have both these characteristics and offer an excellent opportunity to practice a stroke that can be used throughout the body. Full-hand kneading penetrates deeply and oxygenates internal tissues while squeezing out acidic wastes. You will return to this movement often as you massage a pregnant woman.

The hands turn in opposing circles when you knead. If you are right-handed, begin by making a counterclockwise circle with that hand, closing the thumb and forefinger each time you reach the extreme left-hand position of the circle. The two fingers should spread wide open at the opposite side of the circle. On soft tissues, like the buttocks, pick up a fold of flesh each time the thumb closes against the forefinger. When kneading a hard-muscled calf, you won't find much flesh to pick up easily. There it's sufficient to press your thumb into the muscle as you circle. Once you feel comfortable doing that with your right hand, begin circling with the left hand in the opposite direction, picking up flesh with your thumb in the extreme right position and opening the thumb and forefinger on the extreme left side. Put these two movements together, and you're doing a simple and very effective full-hand kneading stroke.

The hands work closely enough to allow each hand to circle in and pick up flesh inside the open thumb and forefinger of the other. Knead in smooth, even circles, avoiding jerky lines or hesitations that will break your rhythm.

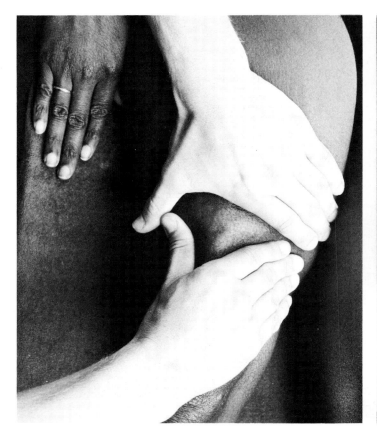

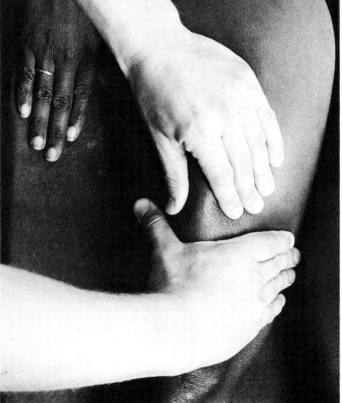

Fingertip Kneading the Hand and Arm

Grasp the forearm exactly the same way you did the palm, but use less pressure here to accommodate exposed blood vessels. Knead from the elbow to the wrist, using wider circles to cover the whole surface of her forearm in a single pass.

If your partner's palm appears swollen, she may be retaining fluids in her extremities, a condition, known as edema, that's fairly common during early pregnancy. Excessive swelling requires medical attention, but minor puffiness can usually be reduced quickly by extended fingertip kneading movements up and down the arm. Whether or not swelling is evident, she is likely to enjoy the extra attention.

Wrap your fingers around the back of your partner's hand for support, and grasp the palm side with the full flat surface of both thumbs. Whenever possible during fingertip kneading, keep the whole flat surface of your thumb, from ball to tip, in contact with her body. Try to avoid digging in with the tips of your thumbs. Concentrate on the fleshy base of her hand, but be sure to move your thumbs around so the entire surface of her palm is covered.

When you're through massaging a woman's palm, stroke each finger once, slowly, from base to tip, and move up onto her forearm. You can continue fingertip kneading up toward the shoulder by modifying your support system for the arm. It's important to elevate the top of the arm in order to reach around it as you knead. To leave both hands free for kneading, tuck her hand under your armpit (fingers flat), and press it close to your body while massaging. A pregnant woman will appreciate the feeling of contact and closeness when her hand is supported by your body. Knead onto her shoulder as far as possible without breaking contact under the arm with your support fingers. The powerful deltoids at the shoulder are used in almost every arm movement. You can begin massaging them from below while kneading the upper arm and finish off during a complete head massage (see page 69).

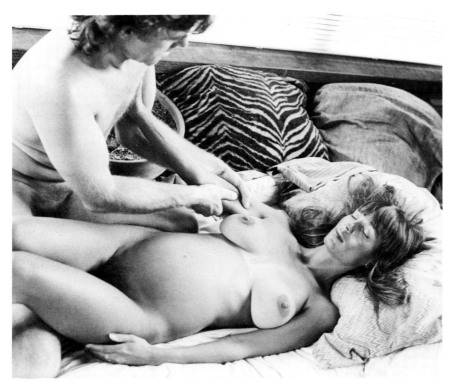

Rotate your thumbs, but keep them pressed together. Allowing the tip of one thumb to rise while the other falls permits you to make two circles at once.

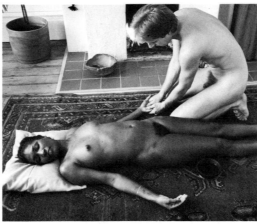

Fingertip Kneading the Perineal Body

Most of the tissue stretching when a baby is born occurs just below the lower end of the vagina, where five muscle groups from the legs, buttocks, and lower back converge on a small fibrous mass called the perineal body. The cut made during an episiotomy permits extra stretching room for this area. Regular massage of the perineal body and the muscles that meet there may make an episiotomy unnecessary.

Use pillows to elevate your partner's midsection while she lies on her stomach with her legs apart. Later on in pregnancy you can use other positions that seem more comfortable to her. Begin with plenty of fingertip kneading to the perineal body between the vagina and the anus. Then focus your attention on the five converging muscle groups that will be stretched during the birth. To keep them supple, massage the area where they originate as well as the perineal body meeting point. Knead the inside top of your partner's thigh all the way back to the bony tip of the sacrum at the base of the spine. Use light friction over the sacrum; then knead the inside top of her other leg. The buttocks offer the best opportunity for full-hand kneading anywhere on the body. Here you can use the whole surface of your hand from the base of the palm to the fingertips. Add extra oil, if necessary, while you pick up handfuls of flesh. You may find that it's possible to pick up more flesh on the buttocks by closing your thumb against all four opposing fingers instead of only the forefinger. The perineal region is supplied from above by a single nerve and its companion artery. Finish off massage of this area by stimulating circulation, indirectly, with a series of fast hand-over-hand strokes on the backs of your partner's thighs.

Regular fingertip kneading of the perineal body and surrounding muscles will keep the whole area supple during the birth.

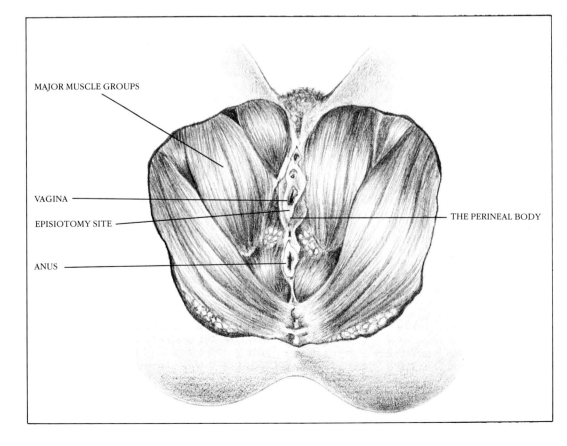

MAJOR MUSCLE GROUPS

VAGINA

EPISIOTOMY SITE

ANUS

THE PERINEAL BODY

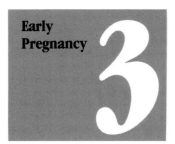

Extra Pressure and Extra Pillows

As a woman learns to relax with massage, she will begin appreciating the most subtle variations in your technique. You might try including the backs of her arms in your back massage or, using both hands, discover a new way to circle the knees. The front of the foot can be massaged from either side of the body, and so can her hands. Discoveries like these mark the beginning of a personal massage technique, which will evolve slowly as you gain confidence. Each new massage stroke becomes an *experience* for a woman, who slowly begins to identify your unique personal style. She learns to recognize the way you touch her arm after you've finished a favorite stroking movement and the texture of your hands during kneading.

One of the variations you may want to consider in early pregnancy is increased pressure, an option that will become difficult in just a few months. As her body begins to change, a woman will usually welcome deep strokes that penetrate to the interior tissues. Try them on thickly muscled parts of the body, like the upper back and legs, where a little feedback from her will indicate whether this is something you want to include in future massages. If it is, the time has come to indulge your imagination and think about pillows.

The idea of extra nonessential pillows brings to mind the sort of indolent, almost sinful luxury that's usually reserved for royalty and libertines. This is exactly what most people want but can never seem to justify having. Deep-stroke massage movements supply you with the justification to indulge your wildest pillow fantasies (budget permitting). There are very few objects of any size or price that will give you as much sustained physical satisfaction as a good pillow.

Happily you can find ample justification for extra pillows at almost every point in a full body massage. If you're massaging on a fairly thin surface, you'll need the cushioning effect whenever you push down firmly. But even on a well-padded massage surface your partner will welcome the extra support of pillows under each shoulder during upper back massage, particularly if her breasts are sore. Use pillows to make a pregnant woman supremely comfortable. She'll appreciate the extra care and attention all through a massage. Moderate size pillows fit nicely under the small of the back and behind the knees while smaller pillows are useful just above the ankle (on each side of the leg) and behind the neck. But why stop there? Real pillow lovers will appreciate tiny pillows (or rolled towels) that support the wrists just enough to allow the hands to go completely limp while they're being massaged. Huge body-size pillows encourage people to collapse and surrender, first to the pillow and then to the massage experience.

Remember that you do need a certain amount of control to be effective in massage. When the two of you begin drowning in a pillow, it's too big for anything but fun.

If you're making your own large pillows remember that foam rubber collapses and becomes completely useless in a few years. Various synthetic fillings are more reliable but the old style down pillow is still best.

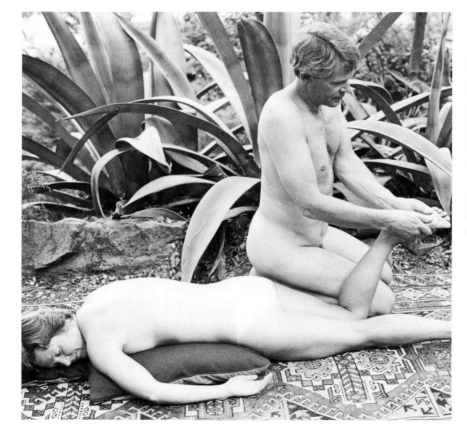

Split Kneading

With a few pillows on hand you're ready to try some deep-pressure massage strokes. These somewhat specialized movements work best on the thighs and across the top of the back, where thick muscles prevent you from pressing down onto a bone. The amount of pressure you use will vary and usually depends on the muscle thickness of your partner's legs. If they are very thinly muscled, this stroke probably won't be suitable. The best way to proceed is to test the movement by pressing down with the flat part of your knuckle. You should feel muscle, not bone, under your fingers. While you press down carefully, a little feedback from your partner will give you a good sense of what feels good. And the next time you won't have to ask.

Split kneading combines ordinary full-hand kneading with a high-pressure closed-fist circling stroke. Use your kneading hand to pick up flesh with the thumb in the usual way while the closed-fist hand presses deeply into interior muscle tissue. Circle with both hands in the same pattern as full-hand kneading. This time, however, the fist hand remains closed and maintains a uniform pressure throughout the stroking cycle.

If you've decided to try split kneading on the thighs, reach across and massage opposite the leg (as shown). This makes it easy to concentrate on the top and outside surfaces of the leg. Ease up on the inside of the thigh, where pressure on the exposed femoral artery can cause problems (see page 100). Your open hand works exactly the same way it did in full-hand kneading (see page 57), opening and closing rhythmically and picking up some flesh with the thumb each time it closes. Close your other hand, and press down into your partner's muscle with the flat part of the middle knuckles. Turn the fist until it faces the open forefinger of the other hand. While you knead in the normal way with your open hand, the fist will press down and circle. When you reach the open thumb position, the fist can circle in until it almost touches the other hand (as shown). One hand opens and closes while it circles; the other circles and presses down into the interior tissues. Use the whole flat surface of your knuckles to circle, and gradually let both hands move down onto the side of your partner's leg. On the leg, this stroke is most effective in the area between the hip bone and the knee. Knead up and down the leg until you've covered that whole area thoroughly. Women who enjoy split kneading (particularly dancers and runners) can't seem to get enough of it.

You can vary the pressing part of the stroke by bringing the whole surface of your hand from knuckle tip to the base of the palm into contact with your partner's leg. Once you've established the right pressure, there's no reason not to go on repeating this movement for a while.

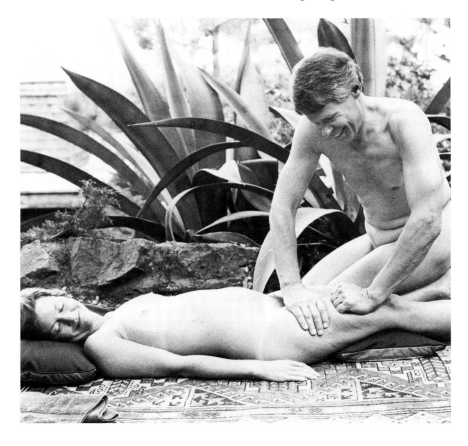

Self-Love and Toe Care

During massage your partner must care enough about herself to enjoy feeling things with every part of the body. Curiously, some people have trouble doing this. A woman who sees pregnancy as nothing more than a troublesome unattractive period has developed so negative a self-image that she is likely to resist any kind of lasting physical pleasure. Pleasure censorship, like insomnia, anxiety, and other purely mental sources of distress, will eventually damage the body as stress levels climb relentlessly. Masseurs solve the problem by working through the body, not through the mind, to reverse the degrading effects of stress. If your partner seems to resist head and back massage, try introducing her to a new experience where the pleasure censorship reflexes may not operate so readily: a complete foot massage that includes all ten toes.

Rediscovering the feet as a source of great sensual pleasure is one of the most delightful surprises of any first full body massage. Feet take an enormous amount of punishment as they are relentlessly tortured by the whims of cruel fashion.

Farthest from the heart and brain, most of the time the feet either ache or feel nothing at all. Once your partner has begun to experience pleasant sensations on her feet, she will realize that each toe is capable of independent feeling. Massage liberates the toes from the tyranny of modern shoes and may permit a woman to enjoy this part of her body for the first time in years.

The notion that toes actually have individual needs may seem frivolous, especially to a woman who automatically resists physical pleasure. Since your partner is likely to benefit so much from a good foot massage, it's sometimes helpful to say a few words before beginning simply to calm her down. (Remember that massage is a nonverbal experience, and any kind of debate will distract her.) It may be useful to point out how the maintenance of expensive possessions can become far more time-consuming than the maintenance of the human body. How does the new car feel? Fine. And how do the new leather-covered seats feel after they've been rubbed down by hand? Soft but still dead. Though they are insignificant and small, each toe is a living

Begin the toe massage by pulling up the sides of each toe with two fingers. You can then grasp the toes, one at a time, and rotate them several times in each direction. Try stroking them along the top or bending all five at once over the edge of your index finger with the flat side of your other hand. Finish by half circling each toe as you pull off it in a spiral pattern.

Ask your partner if she can remember the last time anybody touched her toes. There is nothing to compare with the wonderfully pampered feeling of a foot massage that stops to consider the individual needs of each toe.

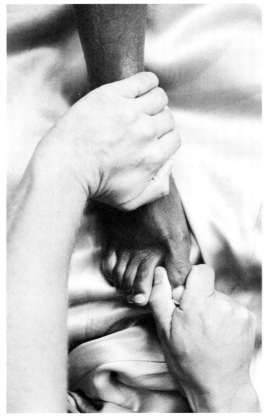

part of you. No matter how much rubbing, polishing, and cleaning you lavish upon any one of your possessions, none of them will ever achieve this status. Don't you, any part of you, deserve better treatment than an object?

Toes can be lifted, rotated, pulled (gently), stroked, squeezed, and cork-screwed. If it's your partner's first experience with massage, she's likely to take a close interest in your toe technique, so why not give her something to remember? A complete toe massage will start up at the knee, where the muscles that operate the toes begin. Concentrate, first, on kneading the calf muscles; you may want to raise your partner's knee in order to relax them more thoroughly. Just below the most visible part of the calf muscles, the tough, fibrous Achilles tendon, the longest in the body, begins and descends all the way to the arch on the bottom of the foot. Press down into it with fingertip kneading and friction movements. You can usually use fairly strong pressures here because the tendon is so well developed.

Rotate the center of your palm on the back of her heel, and knead the bottom of the foot with

your fingertips. Then wrap your hands around the sides of her foot so that your thumbs rest on top and the other four fingers press up into the sole. From this position you can knead the whole top of the foot, then move slowly to her neglected toes. Like fingers, toes are most sensitive along their sides. Whatever you decide to do with your partner's toes, it's important to be consistent on all ten of them. Once she has begun feeling things with her toes, each one becomes sensitive and terribly important.

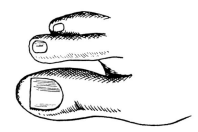

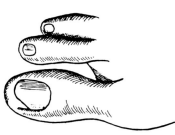

Badly trimmed toe nails will eventually create painful problems that no masseur can correct.

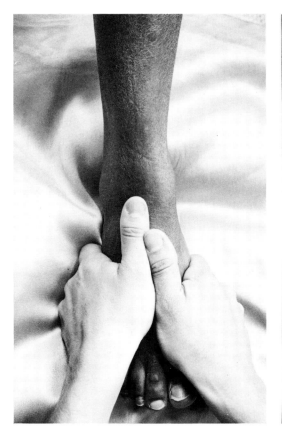

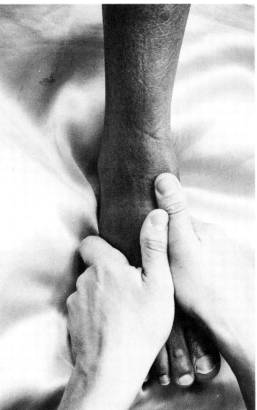

When you're kneading the top of the foot it's easy to move your thumbs up onto the front of the leg. Just above the bone you can feel the tibialis anterior muscle which is involved in the familiar athletic "shin splints" injury. Wrap your fingers around the back of the lower leg and spend an extra minute doing fingertip kneading if your partner is an athelete.

3

Quick Energy with Percussion

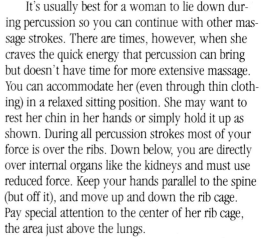

Every thirteen seconds the entire blood supply of the body passes through the lungs, where fresh oxygen is absorbed while waste gases are expelled. The exchange takes place in semipermeable air sacs which are richly supplied with blood vessels and capillaries. Effective respiration depends on good blood circulation within the tissues of the lungs.

Protected on all sides by the rib cage, the lungs cannot be directly influenced by most massage movements. Percussion movements, which transmit vibration all the way through the torso, are a notable exception. Deep-penetrating effects would appear to require a great deal of force, but fortunately percussion movements call for restraint instead of power. A few minutes of percussion will triple the blood supply to a woman's lungs and shake loose internal debris that inhibits breathing. Oxygen levels climb throughout the body and leave her feeling refreshed, as though she had taken a long walk. Enhanced lung power is particularly helpful during pregnancy because the diaphragm, the muscle that controls breathing, is restricted by the growing womb (see page 109).

Begin by cupping your hands to break the force of each tapping contact with your wrists. In all percussion movements your hands should be snapped from the wrist to avoid pounding on your partner's back with the full force of a descending forearm. This wrist-snapping motion will produce a light popping sound as your cupped hands make contact with her back.

It's usually best for a woman to lie down during percussion so you can continue with other massage strokes. There are times, however, when she craves the quick energy that percussion can bring but doesn't have time for more extensive massage. You can accommodate her (even through thin clothing) in a relaxed sitting position. She may want to rest her chin in her hands or simply hold it up as shown. During all percussion strokes most of your force is over the ribs. Down below, you are directly over internal organs like the kidneys and must use reduced force. Keep your hands parallel to the spine (but off it), and move up and down the rib cage. Pay special attention to the center of her rib cage, the area just above the lungs.

You can vary the cupping movement without sacrificing any of its effect by closing your fists and rapping on her back with the flat part of your middle knuckle. Whenever your partner wants extra attention over a single spot, lay one hand flat and tap on the back of your closed fingers with the fist of your other hand. Percussion strokes can extend all the way up onto her shoulders. Near the neck aim for the fleshiest tissues and stay off her bony shoulder blades.

Practice controlling your tapping intensity and rhythm until you can do percussion sequences without thinking about either. A slow, consistent rhythm has a hypnotic effect and will serve your partner better than flashy speed bursts that cannot be sustained. Take it easy, and percussion strokes will work the first time. Use them to relax a pregnant woman who's in a hurry and to introduce shy people to the joys of massage.

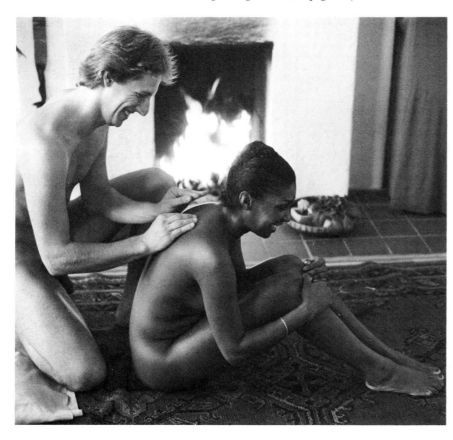

The Full Body Lift

The full body lift is an excellent passive exercise for the complex joints of the lower back. It will stretch tight intervertebral ligaments as well as a variety of lower-back muscles and tendons. A well-executed full body lift will give your partner an unexpected thrill and create the trust you will need to experiment further with passive exercises on the arms and legs.

Since much of your partner's body will be airborne at the climax of this movement, it's important not to drop her. Steady yourself by bracing your body in a tripod position with one foot flat and the knee raised while the other knee is down. Reach behind the arc of her lower back, and clasp your fingers together basket-style. Once you're comfortable and well balanced, lift slowly; sudden, jerky movements will spoil the effect. Elevate her lower back until just the hips and shoulders are in contact with your massage surface. Hold that top position for a few seconds; then lower your partner slowly, the way you raised her. Keeping your hands in place, rest until you're ready to do another back lift. The tripod lifting position takes most of the

effort out of this stroke, and you should be able to repeat it several times.

Arms and legs, which can be elevated from the wrist or ankle, are even easier to lift. Once raised, they can be turned or pulled gently. If your partner gets excited about the full body lift, you can elevate these four other parts of her body while she relaxes and does nothing at all.

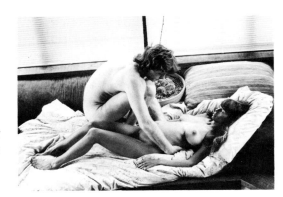

Most joints move in irregular circles. When you encounter resistance back off and work just inside the point of tension. Frequent massage will keep the ligaments, the fibrous bands that connect bones to each other, supple.

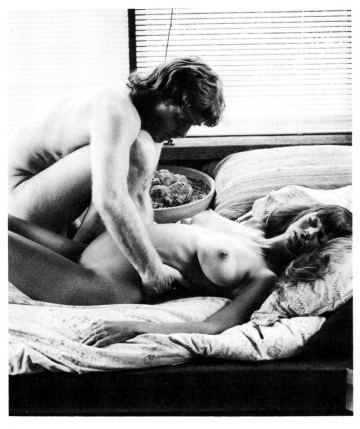

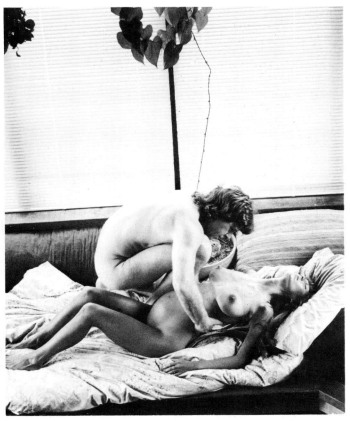

Team Massage

The best people to choose for team massage of a pregnant woman are those who care as much about her as you do. A good professional masseur is always helpful and pleasant, but being well massaged by several people who love you is one of life's most delicious experiences. You can arrange for relatives to participate when they visit, and prospective grandparents are often eager to help. Begin by demonstrating a simple full-hand friction movement that requires no oil. Say a few words about the importance of repetition, and direct the new masseur to a well-muscled calf or hip for practice.

Once your student is comfortable with the friction movement, you can introduce circulation and kneading strokes for the limbs. Each of you can massage a leg with identical movements during early pregnancy, but in late pregnancy, when the side lying position becomes necessary for your partner, it's best to separate and work on different parts of the body. Simultaneous head and foot massage is a rare pleasure that can be experienced by a woman only during team massage.

Whatever you decide to do, be sure to keep your rhythms consistent and maintain contact with your partner's body. Add new movements when you feel the new masseur is ready to learn more, but don't rush things. It's more important to preserve the delightful sensation of being massaged by two people at once than it is to dazzle a woman with fancy technique. Most people begin their interest in massage after giving (or getting) a first one. Don't be surprised if your relatives go home and begin practicing earnestly on each other.

If your pregnant partner becomes a great fan of team massage (many do), you may want to provide her with this experience frequently. Relatives usually aren't available regularly, but your other children certainly will be, and those who are old enough to walk and talk become intensely curious whenever their pregnant mother is massaged. This is an ideal time to encourage curiosity and teach a child some basic massage. Doing so gets him or her involved in the process of pregnancy (just as it did you) and helps the child accept the new baby. Don't let the vivid fantasy life and wild mood swings of

Children tend to jump squarely into the middle of a massage, improvising furiously, only to abandon their partner completely a few minutes later and wander off, paralyzed with boredom. Take advantage of visually exciting strokes, such as percussion and full-hand circulation, to capture a child's attention. Whenever you create activity by doing more massage, you introduce a new and lively reality to the child.

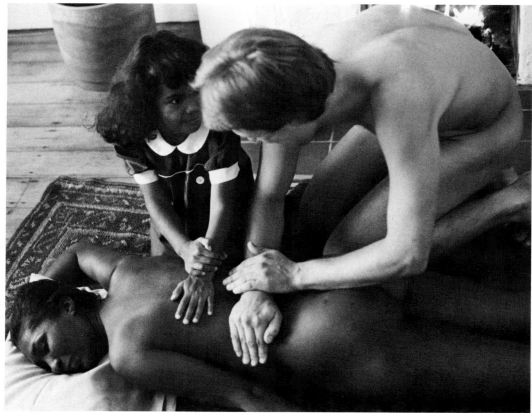

some children be off-putting. Teach the same movements you would to an older relative, and if you're interrupted, try to return to whatever stroke you were doing.

Most children will grasp easily the various techniques used in massage. What bores them is the need to repeat movements and maintain an even rhythm. It helps if you demonstrate how the first stroke in a series sets a rhythmic pattern that subsequent movements must follow. Once that's understood, show the child how massage often supplies a choice when it appears that no choice exists. Demonstrate the various ways a part of the body can be kneaded or stroked; then lift one of your partner's limbs while your child kneads it. Suddenly the child is part of a team and doing an important job.

Point out to your child how content her mother becomes when the two of you massage together. Children cannot easily recognize the difference between deep relaxation and sleep, but they will always enjoy making a contribution during pregnancy.

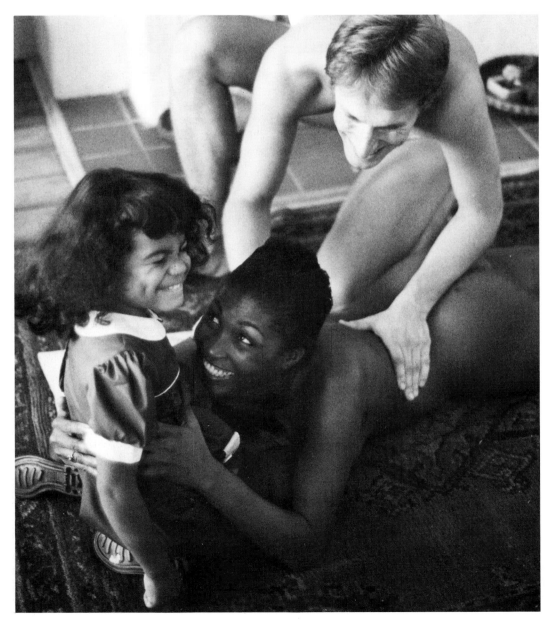

When a child's contribution is obviously appreciated, the room may explode with shouting and laughter. That, of course, marks the end of the team massage; but your child will be back for more, and so will her pregnant mother.

A COMPLETE HEAD MASSAGE

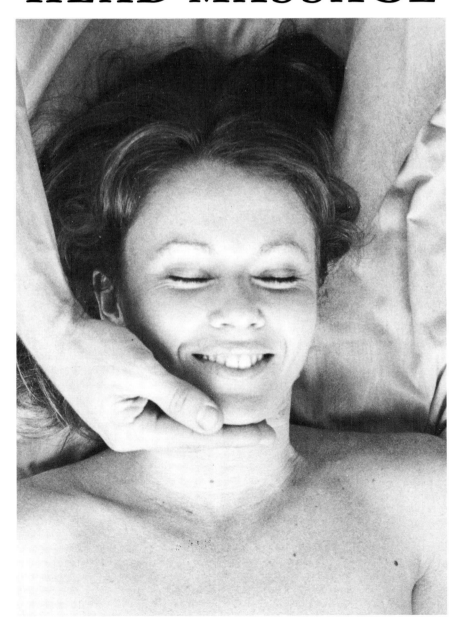

Headaches and the Vasoconstriction Effect

One of the very first changes to occur in early pregnancy is an increase in maternal blood volume to provide for the future needs of the fetus. As blood volume increases, the heart rate, which will fluctuate throughout a pregnancy, speeds up. Both changes can lead to congestion in the brain's internal vascular system, where tiny capillaries have trouble adapting to new demands, thus causing headaches. Eventually, as the elastic blood vessel walls begin to expand and the heart slows down, her headaches will subside. Unfortunately the adaptation process may go on for weeks while a pregnant woman is left to the mercy of throbbing headaches that begin at dawn and may come and go all day. Nothing is more certain to completely undermine her peace of mind and turn pregnancy into a terrible ordeal. Before she reaches for the Tylenol (aspirin can cause blood coagulation difficulties during pregnancy and should not be used), try massaging her head and neck.

Most problems within the brain will manifest themselves as pain behind the eyes, at the temples, or across the forehead. There are direct nerve connections between every internal organ and the surface of the body. Usually disturbances within an organ will be felt on the skin just above it. Exceptions to this rule involve the heart, where pain is transmitted to the left arm, and the diaphragm, where irritation appears around the right shoulder. In both cases the surface sensation, known as "referred pain" because it's so far removed from the source, still indicates a disturbance that originates in an internal organ. This is an especially important concept to consider when you are dealing with a headache because the brain itself is entirely anesthetic. Check carefully with your partner. The area where she actually feels the pain is the best place for you, as a masseur, to vanquish it.

Some of the most painful headaches are caused by stress. Whenever people are under pressure, irritated nerves cause the whole vascular system to contract while the heart beats faster. Most body secretions decrease, blood rushes away from the skin's surface, adrenaline is squirted into the veins, and muscles tighten up all over the body. This built-in phenomenon, known as vasoconstriction, allows mammals to fight the moment something threatening happens.

During stress the normal body priorities are changed. Nervous awareness and muscle tension become more important than good circulation or digestion. For most of our closest relatives in the animal kingdom, stress reduction is merely a question of tearing each other to pieces or carrying on as though that sort of thing were about to happen at any moment. Then, after a gratifying emotional outburst, the heart slows down, blood returns to the skin, and all body systems return to normal. Pregnant Homo sapiens, who find it inappropriate to bay at the moon when the car won't start, may have to live with constricted blood vessels and a racing heart for hours. And that, of course, is the perfect recipe for a splitting headache.

Fortunately masseurs can usually reverse the vasoconstriction effect by simply soothing the nerves. Blood vessels inside the brain will expand while the heart slows down and blood pressure drops. Whether your partner's headache is caused by increased blood volume or stress, the best way to relieve it is to relax the nerves of the face, forehead, and neck.

Be sure your partner has removed makeup, earrings and contact lenses before you begin massaging her head. It's normal for a bit of harmless vegetable oil to get into her hair while you're stroking.

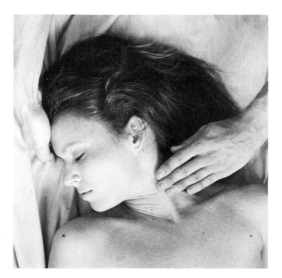

Breaking the Headache Habit

After random pain, headaches are probably the most common symptom of distress in twentieth-century life. If he's not suffering from a headache, modern man is usually busy giving one to somebody else and there's no reason why it should be your partner. She's pregnant and certainly entitled to peace of mind and happiness. With a little bit of quiet time and some warm vegetable oil you can help her get there.

Be careful of massaging a woman who is deeply involved with antiheadache drugs, most of which offer only temporary relief, followed by recurring pain and drug-induced side effects. A masseur who competes with pills may be blamed when the pills fail. Chronic headache sufferers have usually been through the unhappy gamut of chemical pain control often enough to show an interest in a new approach. Offer massage as an alternative, but wait for the effects of the last pill to wear off before you begin. Wait for an hour or two if the drugs were purchased without a prescription, a full day if your partner has graduated to one of the new-age tranquilizers or muscle relaxants which penetrate the brain and alter its internal chemistry. Learn to recognize the effects of these insidious drugs if your partner has been fighting headaches. In minutes all pain passes from her body, and with it most of her identity as an individual human being. A weird rubbery chemical stasis takes over that is usually followed by high anxiety and more pill taking. Offer your partner plenty of water to flush the system, and start massaging when she seems alert once again.

Masseurs should always begin a headache treatment by trying to get a sense of what actually hurts. Tension headaches are usually focused around the forehead and temples; muscle strain, around the back of the skull or on the side of the neck; eyestrain, of course, behind the eyes; and infections, like the flu, are often accompanied by sinus problems with low level and pain throughout the body. People who are trying to quit a legal drug like nicotine, caffeine, or (curiously) aspirin also get headaches. In nearly every case the pain will decline in intensity or disappear completely after a few minutes of head and shoulder massage.

Headaches are distinctly physical problems, but perhaps because they are so clearly stress-related, there's a strong temptation to blame a specific *event* for all the pain. Pregnant women are often encour-aged to "talk it out" with the hope that letting off steam will relieve the tension. Usually this doesn't work because head pain is a good indication that a woman has already reached the point where internal physical changes have occurred. What began as a mental problem has now become a physical one, and masseurs will generally skip the talk, which may bring on even more frustration, and get right to work on the body.

The sequence that follows offers you enough technique to deal with every one of the most common headache situations. If the headache is caused by purely hormonal factors that accompany pregnancy, the relief may be only temporary. Even so, you will be able to substitute hours of peace for hours of anxiety. Stress-related headaches, however, can vanish in minutes, leaving a woman wondering afterward exactly what caused the headache in the first place.

There's no reason to wait until your partner gets a headache to begin using these strokes. They make a superbly relaxing head and shoulder massage, one that she will appreciate often in the months to come. You need only a comfortable place for her to lie down to begin the sequence. Her face and neck can be done without further preparation (like heating the room or undressing). But to cover all the areas that contribute to a headache, it's a good idea to do a complete head massage. The technique for that follows, and if you want something essential and pleasing to offer a woman every day of her pregnancy, it's worth learning all the way through.

A Ten-Minute Complete Head Massage

Many a time I have relieved a tired headache and put a wakeful patient to sleep by ten minutes massage of the head alone, when subsequent applications of longer duration, including both head and body, had no greater effect.

Douglas Graham

Think about massaging a woman, even one you've known for a long time, and you will begin to see her differently. Suddenly the precise size relationship between her head and upper body becomes terribly significant because the head is a large object that must be supported by the muscles below. You learn to look for signs of stress in the muscles of her neck and shoulders and to study the way she carries her head. Understanding this basic body language is very useful in massage.

If your partner has a large head mounted on tiny shoulders, you will need to pay extra attention to her upper back whenever she's massaged. Thick upper-back muscles which are anchored to the skull do most of the work in supporting the head and are usually the first part of a woman's body to register fatigue. The whole shoulder and neck area is a source of almost constant tension for many women, pregnant or not. Add the stress of pregnancy plus a faltering exercise program, and all sorts of unwelcome problems may develop. The muscles can go into spasm, pinching nerves, cutting off circulation to the brain, and torturing a woman

with bouts of excruciating pain. One way to prevent this from happening is to keep her relaxed by massaging the whole head frequently, which takes about ten minutes. Headaches, of course, can last for ten hours.

Begin a complete head massage by relaxing the large muscles of the upper back that support the skull. Massaging neck and skull foundation muscles at the beginning of your headache sequence will make it easier for the smaller muscles of the face and neck to relax when you get to them later. As your partner lies on her stomach, be sure her breasts are comfortable. You may want to add a couple of small pillows under her shoulders for extra support. This will also relieve some of the pressure on the neck when she turns her head to one side. When she is completely comfortable, reach over to the center of the back, and press the full flat surface of your hand across her spine. It is here, beneath the shoulder blades nearly halfway down a woman's back, that your complete head massage will begin.

Add small shoulder pillows if your partner has trouble turning her head all the way to one side. Elevating the shoulders permits her head to turn at a less acute angle or even face straight down. If she prefers the straight down position, which is easiest on a tender neck, use a small pillow to cushion her forehead.

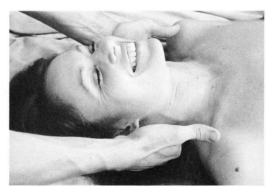

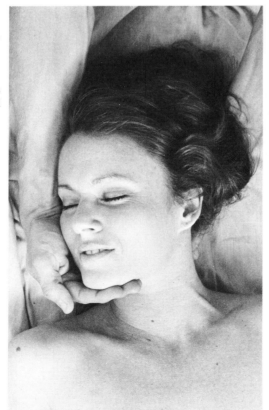

Brain Circulation

In the front of the body most of the blood vessels that supply the brain are well hidden beneath the bones of the upper chest. The long circulation movements that are effective on the muscular limbs are useless here. Pressing down directly on bones accomplishes little and probably won't feel very good to your partner. But on the neck, where the blood vessels are totally exposed, almost any pressure is too much. Masseurs generally avoid the sensitive front of the neck altogether. They turn, instead, to the thickly muscled upper back, where vigorous stroking toward the head will bring oxygen and nutrients to the brain itself.

Before you oil your hands, move your partner's hair out of the way so you can massage her neck later. All the upper-back and shoulder strokes that follow can easily be extended to include the back of the neck, one of the most common places for women to experience tension. A few drops of oil are bound to get into her hair, but don't let that stop you from massaging the neck. Vegetable oil is harmless and can be removed later when she showers.

The muscular upper back, with its protective rib cage around vital organs, will accept more pressure than any other part of the body except the bottom of the feet. Remember to elevate your partner's shoulders with extra pillows so your stroking doesn't put pressure on the abdominal area. Cup your hand slightly so you won't be pressing directly onto her spine, but otherwise make full contact, from the base of the palm to the tips of your fingers throughout the movement.

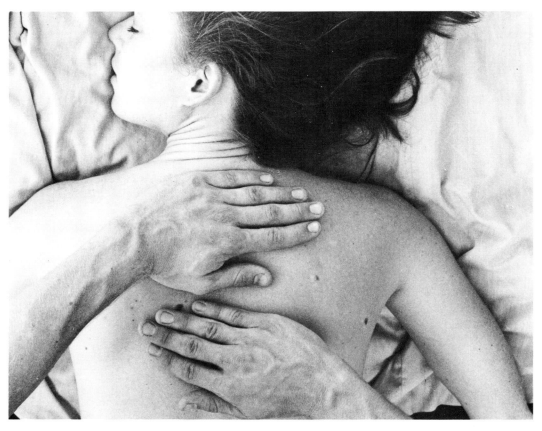

Using moderate pressure, stroke all the way up to the base of her neck with one hand, and then lift it to return to the starting position. The moment you lift your hand, begin up from the center of the back with your other hand. The two hands alternate in this way, stroking up to the base of the neck and returning to the center of the back. Be prepared to add oil if her skin absorbs the first batch you put down.

73

Kneading the Shoulders

Knead with your full hand flat down across the broad muscular expanse just below the neck and with your fingertips across the shoulder tops. The two kneading variations blend nicely as you move across the back. Use as much of your hand as possible and, around the base of the neck, there will be opportunities for one hand to pick up more flesh than the other.

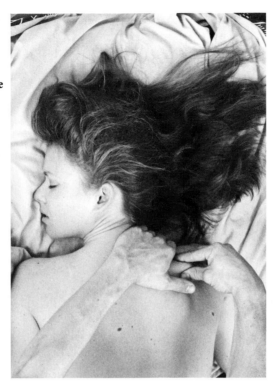

The head is a heavy object that must be supported throughout the day by shoulder and back muscles.

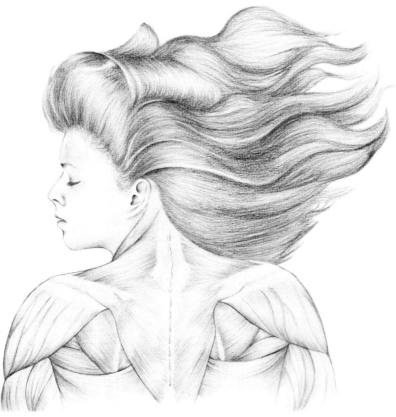

Few strokes anywhere on the body will give a woman more pleasure than kneading the shoulders. This movement will have little effect, however, if your partner is sitting up instead of reclining. It's always best to relax the whole body before massaging any part of it.

Hilary was sitting at the dressing table brushing her hair . . . He moved up behind her, and placed his hands on the back of her neck. He began to work his fingers into Hilary's shoulder muscles. But she did not relax, held her head rigid and averted, so that in the mirror they resembled a tableau of a strangler and his victim. *

Massive upper-back and shoulder muscles that support the head and move the arms will begin to relax only when your partner lies down. Men sometimes have trouble realizing just how much stress this part of a woman's body absorbs every day. The only equivalent area for a man is the lower back, where accumulated stress and exertion can eventually lead to incapacitating cramps. The same kinds of terrible cramps in a woman's upper back can pinch nerves near the shoulder blades, causing terrible headaches. Irritability, a stiff neck, nervousness, even a general sense of exhaustion all can be traced to overly tense shoulder muscles. You really can't spend too much time massaging the shoulders. Relax them, and you convert a woman forever to the joys of massage.

Shoulder kneading calls for two variations on the basic kneading stroke, the hands turning in opposing circles as you knead. As they turn, the space between the forefinger and thumb opens and closes. Each time it opens, move into the gap created with your other hand, and pick up a fold of flesh (as shown). The two hands continue to circle, opening and closing in rhythm and picking up a fold of flesh once every revolution. Whether you're doing full-hand or fingertip kneading, be sure to lift that fold of flesh with your *thumb* each time you circle.

---

*David Lodge, *Changing Places,* (Harmondsworth, Middlesex, England: 1975), Penguin Books, Ltd., pp. 204–205.

Shoulder Friction

Pain, tension, and irritability are often related to tightness in a muscle, a condition you can easily feel. And when you feel it, there's no better quick solution than a few minutes of deep friction. If your partner's shoulders ache, don't hesitate to begin a complete head massage with this movement. See if you can find out exactly where the pain is, and start by pressing down directly over the tender area. If it's too sensitive for direct pressure, simply back off and work nearby. Most of the time direct pressure on fatigued muscles is very welcome. Don't be surprised if you hear your partner moan with pleasure as you begin.

Friction strokes are most effective without oil. If you're working on already oiled skin, remember to press down so your friction hand turns on your partner's muscles, not on the surface of her skin.

It's far better to prolong low-frequency friction for several minutes than to begin with an intense flurry that cannot be sustained for more than a few seconds. Push down while you turn. Sometimes, after a few minutes, you can actually feel tensed shoulder and neck muscles begin to soften. And what your partner feels then is blessed peace— perhaps for the first time in months.

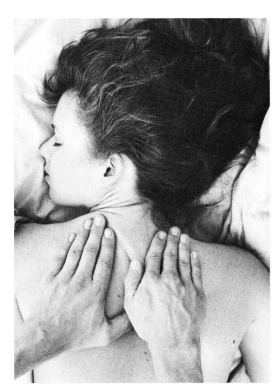

Every friction stroke should be anchored so the vibration effect remains local. Use your left hand as an anchor hand which will stabilize her head and back while you rotate evenly on her shoulder with the whole surface of your right hand. Use your fingers to concentrate pressure on the tops of the shoulders (as shown). Be sure to choose a pressure and a frequency of rotation that feel comfortable to both of you.

Fingertip Friction to the Sternomastoid and Neck

Hold her neck with four fingers of each hand allowing a small gap between your fingertips to avoid the spine. Rotate your hands in small opposing circles pressing up as you go. When one hand is up the other should be down but both hands remain in contact with your partner's neck. After circling for a minute or more, you begin to notice a remarkable difference in the way her neck feels. Hard muscle bound tissue softens, the head falls back as it should and finally, her expression is altered. Where a certain tautness that one associates with high anxiety once prevailed you see tranquility and peace.

Fingertip friction is useful in reaching tiny crevices, bulges, and connections where the full hand simply will not fit. Rather than ignore a tiny spot at the beginning of one of the body's major muscles, why not massage it? While you're working on the back of your partner's body, it's easy to reach the back of her ear, source of the noble sternomastoid muscle, used in almost every head movement. You'll return to this muscle after she has turned over, when it appears as the familiar arc that sweeps down from the skull to the shoulder blade whenever her head is turned.

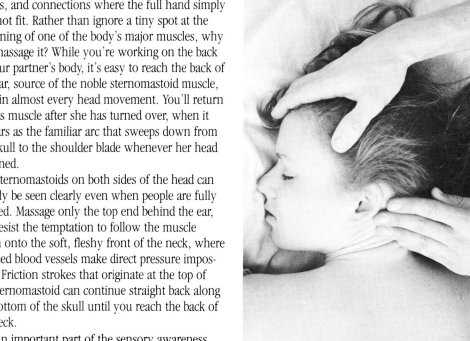

Sternomastoids on both sides of the head can usually be seen clearly even when people are fully dressed. Massage only the top end behind the ear, and resist the temptation to follow the muscle down onto the soft, fleshy front of the neck, where exposed blood vessels make direct pressure impossible. Friction strokes that originate at the top of the sternomastoid can continue straight back along the bottom of the skull until you reach the back of the neck.

An important part of the sensory awareness process you work with in massage is introducing people to new sensations—one at a time. This modest stroke allows you and your partner to explore the backs of her ears and the base line of the skull. Most people have trouble remembering the last time anyone touched them there.

No part of the body responds so dramatically to massage as the back of a woman's neck. Once you've massaged the shoulders (always do that first) a thorough neck massage will delight her.

While you're massaging the back of her neck be sure to reach up with two fingers of each hand to the top center tissue just below the skull. Here, where the brain meets the spine, you can feel the same softening as you rotate and press up in opposing circles with your fingertips.

Turning Over

Turning over is the only thing you ever ask your partner to do during a massage. Try to make the transition as smooth as possible. A word or two whispered in her ear or a prearranged sound (like a musical tone) will do.

If she's been under pressure lately, tensed upper-back muscles probably made turning the neck difficult and caused her scalp to tighten. Now that you've massaged these muscles, she may notice an immediate improvement the moment she begins to turn her head. Many women have resigned themselves to accept constant tension around the shoulders as the price that must be paid for a hard day's work. They begin to worry only when the effects of accumulated tension reach the muscles of the face. Unfortunately nervously dabbing worry lines with expensive creams and jellies accomplishes little if the muscles of the neck and shoulders are near spasm. You've taken the first step in a complete head massage by relaxing these muscles. Her face may already look more relaxed even though you haven't touched it yet.

Touch the center of her forehead and make yourself comfortable while she settles down. Check to be sure your oil is nearby. You'll need just a few drops on your fingertips to massage the delicate interior muscles of the face.

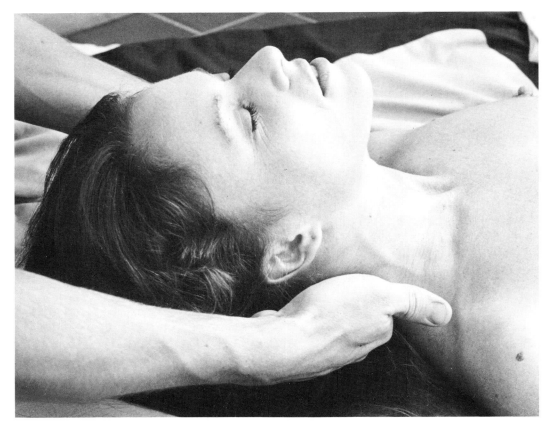

Some women enjoy the extra feeling of support from small rolled pillows behind the neck, in the small of the back and behind the knees. Without interrupting the massage or opening her eyes your partner can tell you exactly where they need to be placed.

Testing for Tension in the Neck and Shoulder Muscles

Relaxed neck and shoulder muscles are such an important prerequisite for successful facial massage that it's useful to perform a simple tension test before you begin on the face. Your reminder before the massage started, on how you would do all the work lifting and turning her limbs, comes in handy here. Your partner will now understand that she doesn't need to help whenever a part of her body is moved. Any help you do get will be involuntary and a sign of tension in the surrounding tissues.

As you massage around the body, there are several easy tests you can do to find out just how relaxed your partner has become. One of the best is to lift the neck with both hands and allow her head to fall back slowly. Reach behind her neck, and cup your hands (as shown), leaving a space for her spine to pass between your fingertips. Lift slowly and evenly on the back of her neck; be sure not to jerk her body. As you lift, the position of her head will tell you just how relaxed she feels around the neck and shoulders. If the head remains upright, you can be certain the neck and shoulder muscles are still tense. You may want her to turn over once

again so you can massage the upper back and neck some more. This is an extra step for both of you, but it's worth the trouble if you want to be effective on the face. You can often feel a tangible softening in tensed muscles when you massage them a second time. After a while repeat the tension test. When the muscles of the neck and shoulders are fully relaxed, her head will fall back (as shown) when you lift her neck.

When you find tension anywhere in the body, massage the surrounding area and remain silent. Lecturing your partner about how nervous she seems will intensify her discomfort and may make the whole massage an unpleasant experience. Her tension is involuntary, and so is the relief she will feel when you're through massaging the head and neck.

Correct hand position (beneath the neck) for the tension test.

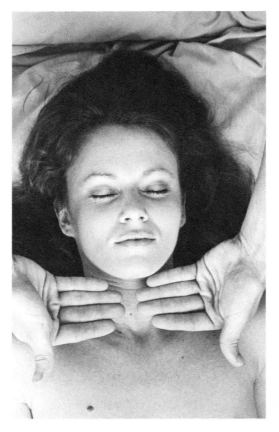

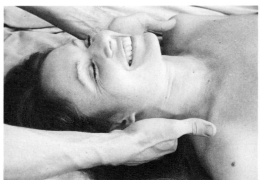

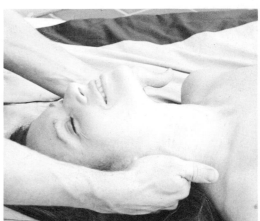

Pulling the Head

During massage the neck and shoulder muscles can be relieved of their burden in carrying the head. In fact, you can go one step farther and reverse all the force normally exerted by gravity when you pull away from the head. Human beings must have been designed with a certain amount of pulling and stretching in mind because everywhere you need to pull on the body there seems to be a set of natural handles. On the skull you'll find them at the back of the head, where the skull indents to meet the neck, and at the chin.

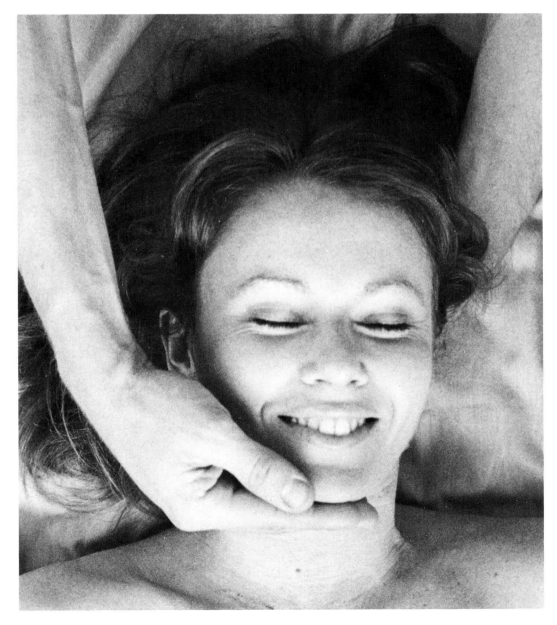

Grasp the back of the skull with the side of your forefinger and middle finger and hold the chin as shown. Pull back evenly; the chin should remain level. Once you've put some tension on the skull, hold it for half a minute while you turn her head at the chin from one shoulder to another.

Pressing the Face and Pressing the Forehead

Simply being held increases a woman's sense of security and allows her to begin feeling things with her face. This is a good time to dispel the misplaced notion that bony parts of the body, like the head, hands, and feet, are somehow less tactile than fleshy areas. You can help her enjoy feeling things with her face by carefully inserting the tips of your little fingers into her ears while you press. As each sense is attenuated (sight and now sound), her tactile sense will grow more acute.

The sumptuous forehead press, the centerpiece of every head massage, can vanquish a headache in less than one minute. Experienced masseurs have seen this happen so often that it no longer comes as a surprise when a single movement accomplishes more than a whole bottle of pills.

During this movement you compress the whole surface of the forehead, and your partner immediately feels a profound sense of relaxation. Just millimeters beneath your hands is your partner's brain, where the forehead press is relished. Equalizing the pressure from fingertips to the base of your palm is the secret to making this stroke work for you. You may return to the forehead press several times during a head massage, and each time it will be appreciated.

A forehead press can last for twenty seconds or for several minutes. All you need do is apply pressure; the hands do not move. The first time you try this stroke, a headache may vanish in thirty seconds as you compress swollen forehead nerves. Even if the pain returns, there is almost always a period of relief while you're pressing. The first grateful sigh usually means that more massage elsewhere on the head and neck will send the headache on its way.

Like every massage stroke, the forehead press can be enjoyed just for the wonderful sensation it produces. The center of the forehead, where Buddhists say the third eye is located, is one of the most sensitive spots on the body. Make that spot, just under the center of your bottom hand, the last place you touch at the end of the forehead press. Lift the edges of your hand slowly. Then break contact for an instant with the center of your palm (it's the only time you'll do so in massage), and immediately go on to the next movement or to the next forehead press.

Press the sides of your hands against the sides of her face and temples, center the thumbs on her forehead, and squeeze gently. Hold the pressure silently for about a minute; then release it very slowly.

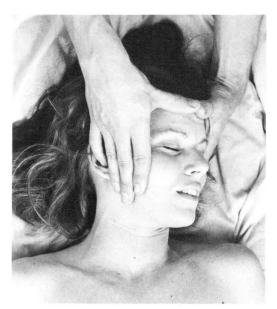

Keep your fingers together, and lay your hands, one on top of the other, across your partner's forehead. Allow both hands to form themselves to the curvature of her head before you use any pressure. To do this effectively, you need only maintain an even contact from your fingertips all the way to the base of your hand. Then press down evenly across the whole surface of your hand.

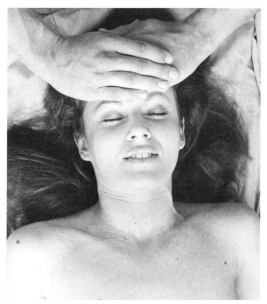

Forehead Friction

Friction anywhere on the face is likely to cause the whole surrounding area to move. That doesn't really present a problem down on the cheeks near the mouth because most people enjoy having their lips pulled into odd shapes for a moment or two. On the forehead, though, poorly anchored friction strokes can put enough pressure on the skin below the eyebrows to force the eyes open. That puts you eye to eye with a very disappointed woman, who must then be coaxed into closing her eyes once again and continuing with the massage. Save yourself the embarrassment by anchoring forehead friction strokes correctly before you begin.

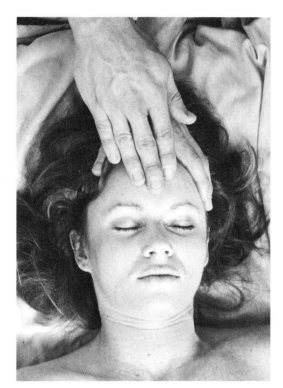

Anchor from above for fingertip friction across the whole surface of the forehead. Spreading your forefinger and thumb, press down gently onto the forehead as you make contact along your partner's hairline. This will tighten skin tension across the surface of the scalp and loosen it over the whole forehead.

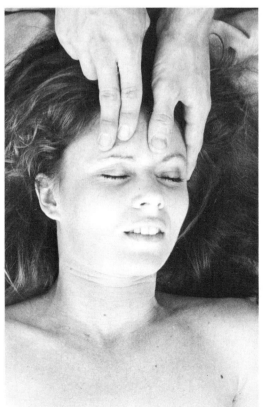

When concentrating a friction stroke on a specific spot, perhaps the source of headache pain, try anchoring from the side of the stroke. That way you can push loose skin directly into the path of your friction fingers. Keep your fingers together, and feel the many contours of the forehead as you work back and forth across it in tiny circles.

Temple Friction and Fingertip Kneading the Face

People enjoy temple friction so much that they will attempt it on themselves. How much better it feels, though, to relax the whole body and let somebody else massage your temples. Like the forehead press, temple friction can be repeated several times in the course of a complete head massage. Return to it after massaging the cheeks, neck, or eyes; each time your partner will relish the sensation.

During temple friction your thumbs remain perfectly still on the center of a woman's forehead while your fingers circle slowly on the temples. On the upper part of the face, movements can be centered in the middle of the forehead by pressing lightly on that spot with both thumbs. This allows you to maintain some pressure on the forehead, balance your hands, and divide your attention evenly. Each side of the face should get equal amounts of pressure and skin contact.

You can vary temple friction by changing the way you circle with your fingers. Rotating in opposing directions is easy enough once you've tried it a couple of times. Whatever kind of circling you choose, be sure it's smooth and rhythmic. Little strokes, in massage, move at the same speed as big ones.

Once again, you are generating pleasure just millimeters away from the brain. Although the brain itself is anesthetic, movements like temple friction reach inside to soothe nerves and relax interior blood vessels.

Wrinkle lines around the eyes and mouth are caused not by imperfect skin but by a general weakening of the underlying muscle tissue. Delicate fingertip kneading strokes will develop muscle tone on the face just as full-hand strokes will condition the back and thighs. A few minutes of kneading will invigorate the muscles, soothes the nerves and empties the tissues of irritating acidic wastes. The latest miracle skin cream or jelly, no matter how expensive, can only sit passively on the surface of the skin until somebody washes it off.

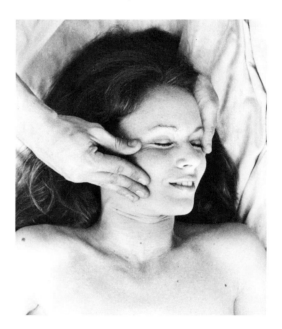

When massaging the cheeks knead with both hands on either side of your partner's face. Up around the eyes it's best to anchor one side of the head (as shown) while you knead the other. Circle with your hand, picking up flesh between the thumb and forefinger once in each revolution. A light oiling is all you need on the face. Kneading the face produces some of the most exquisitely tender moments in massage. Take your time, and let her enjoy it.

Press down on the center of your partner's forehead with your thumbs, and feel for the temples with two or three fingers of each hand. Find the soft depression inside a circle of bone at the corner of the eyes. Press into the depression, fill it with your fingers, and circle gently.

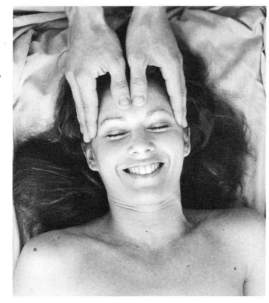

Sternomastoid Friction

If emotional tension has been a persistent problem, look closely at the muscles of the neck to see if any of them have gone into spasm. Nervous tension is always transmitted directly to the muscles, and no muscles anywhere on the body are more closely linked to headaches than the sternomastoids (also called the sternocleidomastoids) on the sides of the neck. These important muscles, first massaged when your partner was on her stomach, are used in rotating, flexing, and even extending the head. Most stiff-neck problems, the usual prelude to chronic

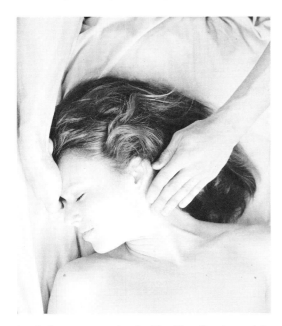

headaches, are associated with either the sternocleidomastoids or the massive trapezius that begins on the back of the skull and mushrooms onto the back. Once either becomes cramped or even strained, any activity more complicated than watching television becomes a real chore.

The sternocleidomastoid has several parts, but the largest is very easy to find and feel. The muscle descends from behind each ear to the front center of the neck and can be seen clearly on each side when the chin faces an opposing shoulder. When you're massaging nearby, rotate your partner's head to one side by grasping it at the chin and behind the skull. As her chin comes around to face one of her shoulders, you will see the sternocleidomastoid appear on the exposed side of the neck (see illustration). Once the muscle has been located, there's a simple test you can do to see if it's in spasm or over-

stressed. Touch it with one hand halfway down the neck, and have your partner turn her head until the chin rests on your hand (see illustration). You should feel the muscle relax completely as it "disappears." If it remains hard or even just firm, you may have found the source of your partner's headache problems: a muscle spasm just below the brain.

Even though the sternomastoid is easy to see, trying to massage its whole length presents some unusual problems. The neck is a very delicate place, with several large exposed arteries that will not accept any kind of deep pressure. Unfortunately that rules out many of the strokes you would use to pump oxygen into cramped muscles elsewhere in the body. Nevertheless, fairly vigorous massage strokes are useful around the top end of the muscle at the edge of the skull. Lower down, around the soft tissues of the neck, you have to be content with light stroking movements that will soothe the nerves.

Perpetually stiff neck muscles here or behind the skull are a clear sign that your partner is under too much pressure. A regular program of general massage, with an emphasis on neck and shoulder strokes, is necessary.

Begin by anchoring your partner's head at the forehead with the full flat surface of your hand, keeping your fingers together. Press down and make small circles on the top of the sternomastoid, the part just behind and below your partner's ear. If the muscle seems tight, turn her head with your anchor hand until the chin is pointed toward the center of the chest. This will relax the muscle, unless it's cramped, and allow you to press in further. Your friction should become lighter as you work down to the halfway point of the muscle in the soft tissues of the neck. Below this point let friction give way to light stroking movements.

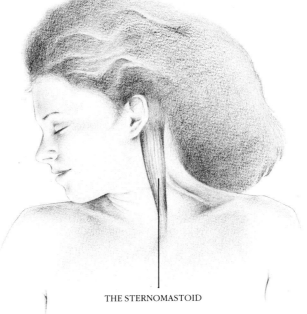

THE STERNOMASTOID

Some headaches are caused by muscle spasms just below the brain.

Stroking the Eyes

Every eye stroke must be anchored on the bone around the eye socket. The contact skin surfaces are so minute that anchoring may only involve steadying the part of the fingers inside the eye socket. Rest part of each finger on the forehead and on the bone just below the eyes. This will absorb any extra pressure caused by a sudden shift in your position or any stresses that reach your fingers. Your fingers can then travel along the bone, making only the slightest contact with her eyelid.

Eyelids are the most delicate structure you will touch during massage. At a fiftieth of an inch the skin of the eyelids is the thinnest anywhere on the body. The slightest pressure will reach the surface of the eye and, from there, penetrate deep into the brain. Very seldom are eyelids intentionally brought into contact with another object. People may have been kissed there for a moment, but they are rarely touched. They seem so delicate that it is sometimes difficult to believe that the eyelids actually *can* be touched by another person. Doing so very lightly will demonstrate to your partner the amazing range of feeling available to her during massage. A tiny bit more pressure will bring on the bizarre intraretinal color bursts known as phosphenes. Eye massage—full of gossamer sensation and strange lights.

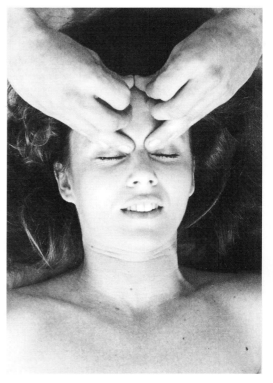

Use all four fingers, one at a time, to stroke the eyes, and keep your thumbs centered on her forehead. Each finger travels along the bony ridge from one end of the eye to the other. The pressure part of the stroke should be up, against the bone, allowing your fingertips to trace the shape of her eyelid. The fingers follow each other across the eye, beginning with the little finger and ending with the forefinger.

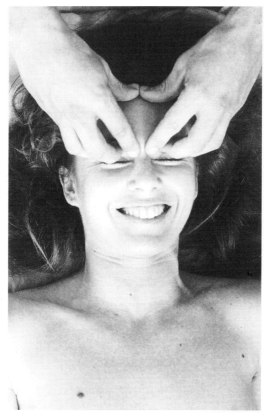

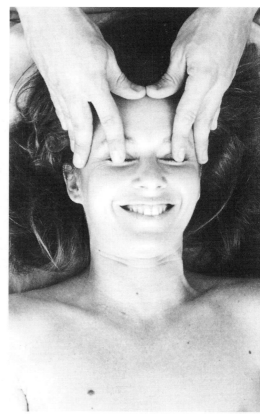

LATE PREGNANCY

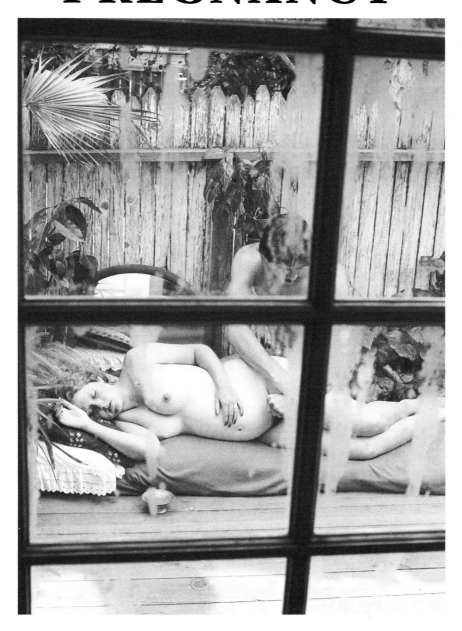

5

Great with child, and longing . . .
for stewed prunes

Shakespeare

To the expectant father whose third trimester wife has just given him this book:

Are you feeling nervous and almost overwhelmed? Are you secretly wondering if these techniques are worth learning? If you've never experienced a massage have somebody give you one. (see p. 130)

When you do a massage, your partner should do absolutely nothing. Even when she's just sitting in a chair, driving, or propped up in bed watching television, all kinds of muscles that need to be relaxed during massage are in use. Normally, if your partner wants to experience massage at its very best, there are really only two choices to consider: Either she relaxes on her stomach, hands at her side, or she rolls over onto her back. Different-size pillows will fit naturally behind the neck, knees, and ankles and under the small of the back to give a kind of total support. Traditional back and stomach positions work so well it seems a great shame to abandon both of them in the later stages of pregnancy, but eventually every woman reaches a point where it's necessary to do so. When she can't lie comfortably on her stomach, even with the extra support of shoulder pillows, it's time for a change. By then her belly has grown large enough to put pressure on abdominal arteries near the spine that bring blood to the legs; and too much time on the back will constrict circulation.

If you want to continue with massage, she must take up the side lying position and stay with it until the birth. Your partner simply reclines on her side with one arm usually draped across her stomach. From there she can move her arms and legs into a number of side lying positions and adjust her whole body to stay comfortable. It allows her some crucial mobility, even so, the change can be so confusing that familiar massage strokes and sequences may become difficult. You knead one side of the body only to find that there's no way to reach over and knead the other. One arm, one foot, or one hand is completely free while the other lies half-buried. Your partner's top arm and leg, no longer held firmly in place by gravity, will tend to fall forward when you do circulation strokes, and in fact, her whole body can roll while you're trying to massage a hip.

Why, then, bother to massage at all in the latter part of pregnancy? One reason is that the benefits available to a woman now, when internal changes have accelerated, are even more impressive than during early pregnancy. More important, your woman may have learned to crave massage and depend on it. Why not give her exactly what she wants?

Look again at the side lying position, and you will realize that it permits you to do new things that were very difficult in the standard positions. And there are ways to adapt nearly all the basic massage movements to it without upsetting your partner. Instead of trying to force your hands under the bottom arm or leg, you can concentrate on a whole side of her body, then have her roll over and massage the other side.

This part of the book will show you how to adapt basic massage to the special needs of late pregnancy.

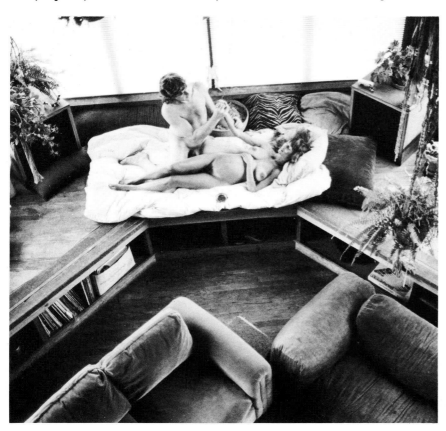

Getting Comfortable in the Side Lying Position

All that fooling around with pillows in early pregnancy was just a rehearsal for the kind of attention your partner needs in her final months. Remember that you are now massaging two people simultaneously, and you need to think of both of them at all times. Every part of the body can still be massaged; you'll just have to stop and let your pregnant partner rearrange herself from time to time.

Be flexible, and the side lying position will work well for your partner on a daily basis. Occasionally she may still want to try lying on her back, although the growing baby will weigh heavily on internal organs and blood vessels to the legs. Soon she will return to the side lying position and rock back and forth a bit until she gets comfortable. Provide her with a well-cushioned massage area (four inches of foam rubber or similar padding) and several pillows for improvising support wherever it's needed. Getting comfortable is really up to the woman, but sometimes (especially during a first pregnancy) she may get confused about where to turn next. When this happens, you can make suggestions (never give orders in massage). Keep your

pillows within reach, and don't hesitate to help by lifting her limbs when she needs to reposition them. She will probably want to move her arms more often than her legs, but whatever limb you're lifting, remember to support it above and below the joint. Move around, before you lift, until you're in a comfortable position to help her with both hands.

A little extra care while you set things up will bring peace more quickly to your partner's restless body. Put oil and towels where they can be reached conveniently but will remain out of the way if she needs to move. Be sure that your massage area will stay warm enough for her and that the two of you will not be disturbed.

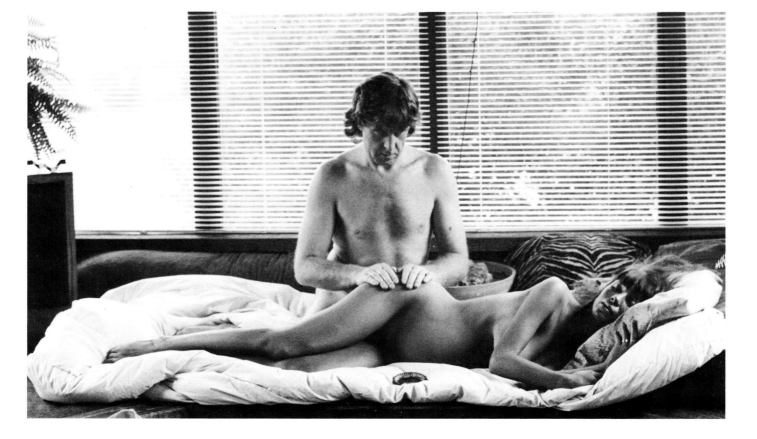

Long Hair in Late Pregnancy

In the side lying position long hair tends to fall against a woman's body and will get very oily when you massage her shoulders. No matter what precautions you take, she's going to pick up some oil in her hair during a massage. (Pinning up the hair makes scalp massage difficult and creates a bulky uncomfortable lump at the back of her skull.) Ordinary vegetable oil is harmless; in fact, it may even do the hair some good. The best way to avoid drenching her with oil is to rearrange the hair before you begin massaging. Be sure to move the

hair yourself rather than ask your partner to assist. Sudden hair combing instructions are bound to be unsettling to a woman who is just beginning to relax.

Arrange the hair the same way you would any other part of the body, using slow, deliberate movements. Don't allow her to get the impression that her hair is simply being tossed aside. A woman is aware of her hair being moved; a little extra care will help convince her that during massage you will be just as attentive to all her needs.

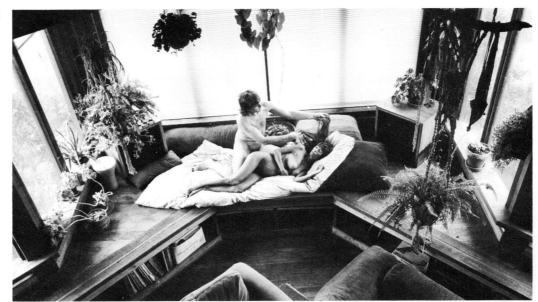

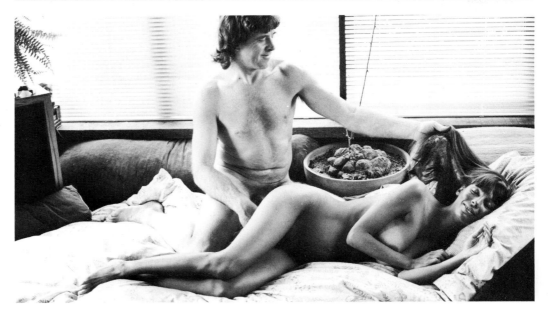

Massaging the Hands and Arms in the Side Lying Position

If you're beginning with massage in late pregnancy, the hands are a good place to start when your partner seems nervous about being touched. Fortunately everyone is accustomed to being touched on the hands by strangers. Massage her hands until she begins to relax; then continue with the arms and torso. Hands are the easiest part of the body to massage in the side lying position. There's no reason to turn your partner since both hands can be massaged from one side of the body. If you are giving your first late pregnancy massage, a few minutes of hand stroking is an easy way to gain confidence before you go on to other parts of the body. All you need do is lift and arrange each arm once, and hand massage can begin without disturbing your partner again.

Be sure her top arm from shoulder to elbow joint is resting along the side of her body so the arm will support itself while you massage. Lift the hand until it's roughly parallel to the rest of her arm. In that position you can hold it with both your hands (as shown), turn it easily, and massage both sides. Occasionally, while you're kneading (but not during fric-

tion or percussion, when downward pressure could be troublesome), you may want to rest the forearm lightly across her belly. Circulation strokes for the arms work best when a woman can lie on her back. When it's not comfortable for her to do this, concentrate on fingertip kneading and light friction movements on the arms.

After massaging the hands and arms, you can conveniently move on to the legs.

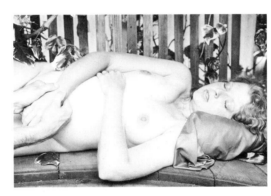

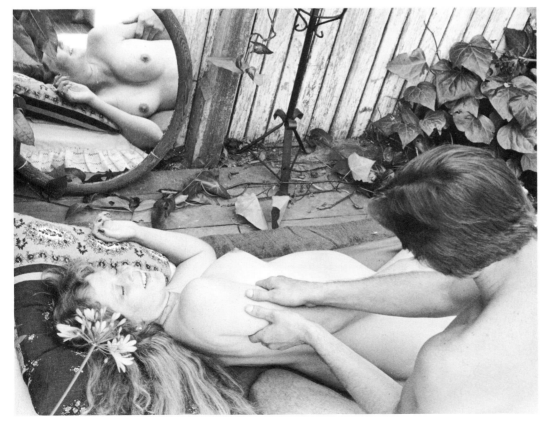

To knead the back of the hand, simply reverse the palm kneading position you used in early pregnancy. Turn the hand palm down, grasp the palm side with four fingers of each hand, and knead the top with the broad flat surface of your thumbs.

Clearing the Lymphatic System

Circulation strokes serve an important double purpose in late pregnancy, when increased abdominal pressure restricts vascular and lymph flow in the legs. It may be essential to your partner's sense of well-being to stroke her legs an extra dozen times every day. This assists the heart in pumping blood through the veins while stimulating the lymphatic vessels, an independent system that carries a milky white fluid called lymph to every part of the body. Good lymphatic circulation strengthens the immune system by bringing antibodies to an infection site and draining toxic wastes from the tissues. These internal effects cannot be as easily isolated and measured as steady vascular blood pressure but are no less essential to good health.

Lymph flow is entirely dependent on the action of local muscles squeezing fluid through the vessels because there is no central organ like the heart to aid circulation. During periods of inactivity the flow tends to stagnate, and wastes accumulate at collection nodes throughout the body (see illustration). This slows muscle recovery rates and contributes to a heavy, congested feeling that oppresses people who lead sedentary lives. Circulation strokes stimulate the lymphatic system and begin the process of removing irritating wastes from the body.

Good lymphatic circulation is one of the most important elements of the extraordinary fluid release effect (see page 44). When ambitious exercise programs become difficult, fluid release massage will release a woman from nagging irritations and leave her legs feeling light and strong. Extra time spent on the legs, particularly the left leg, where the descending colon adds pressure from above, tones the veins and will keep the lymphatic system clear.

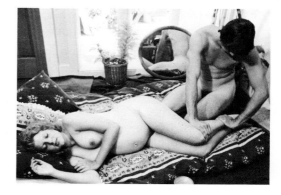

Lymphatic vessels are concentrated in a fine network around the nipples, and wastes and toxins carried by the lymph system are collected in nodes at the edge of the torso.

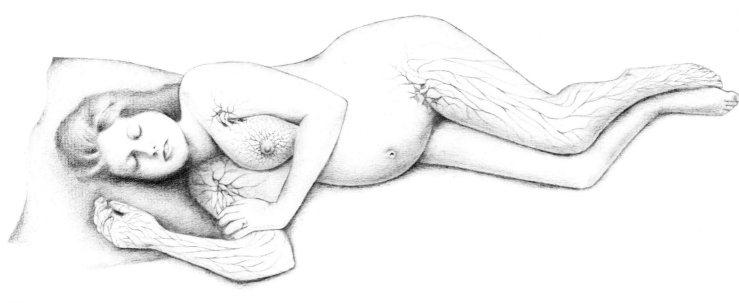

The long circulation stroke you used to push blood through the venous system toward the heart (see page 54) can easily be adapted for use in late pregnancy, when the lymphatic system needs extra attention. While you can't expect your partner to remain on her back for extended periods, it's easy to break the stroke into two sections: one that stops at the knee and one that begins just above the knee and ends at the hip. If you don't mind twisting and turning a bit, you can also press all the way up the side of her leg, bending your hands around the knee. Both variations will permit your partner to continue in the side lying position with her legs bent at the knee.

If you decide to divide your circulation stroke into two parts, it's better to use a separate hand approach, which allows for extra pressure on the leg. Be sure to mold your hands to the changing shape of her legs so there's always contact from the fingertips to the bases of your palms. Most of your pressure should be concentrated on the fleshy sides of her legs. Go easy on the bony fronts of her lower legs and around the knees.

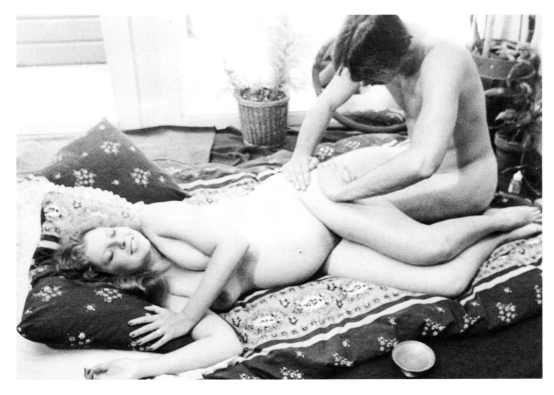

Stroke up to the knee with one hand, and then, as you're returning to the ankle, press up with the other hand. When you've done this ten times, cross over the knee (lightly), and massage the top of the leg the same way.

5

Fingertip Kneading the Leg

Fingertip kneading allows you to massage the intricate web of ligaments and tendons around the body's most complex joint, the knee. Avoid pressing hard on the sides of the kneecap where internal structures will move. Concentrate lower down on the fleshy sides of the knee where the major bones of the leg meet.

Down near the knee you may want to lift her leg (with both hands) and support it on your thigh. The extra support gives your partner a feeling of security and makes it easier for you to reach around the side of her leg.

In the side lying position, a woman's thigh can be kneaded from above or below. If you're interested in massaging every part of her legs and feet, it's better to work from below so you can move up and down her leg freely. The kind of kneading you do depends on the size relationship between your hands and her legs. If your hands are big enough to wrap easily around the lower part of the calf, you can use the thumbs-together technique (see page 58). That's the best, but not the only, way to use fingertip kneading. It's very important, particularly on the thigh, not to squeeze hard on the side of her legs to force your thumbs together. Follow the contour of her leg as it widens out at the thigh, and when it becomes difficult to keep your thumbs together, simply allow them to drift apart. You will still be able to circle with each thumb, but they won't be in constant contact from base to tip. Instead, the thumbs will follow each other at a slight distance, moving in opposing circles as you go up and down her leg. If the two thumbs move in identical circles, you may fall into a scrubbing motion that is much less pleasing than the thumbs-opposed movement. Both thumbs should always be in motion but at opposite ends of their respective circles. Near the hip you may want to change the position of your fingertips to bring the thumbs closer together.

You may also reverse this process and keep your thumbs tightly pressed together while your fingertips glide up from the sides of your partner's leg. Whichever approach you choose, be sure to oil her entire leg before you begin, so your whole hand can go where it needs to go. Once again, be careful not to squeeze hard on the inside of her thigh and the exposed surface of the femoral artery (see illustration, page 100). Light pressure there is best. No matter how you choose to approach this movement, it will be necessary to change your hand position several times. As you move up and down her leg, hand position changes can be smooth and almost effortless, so what you partner *feels* is the surface of your thumbs circling on the muscles.

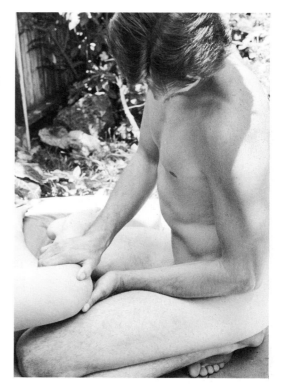

Hot Stroking the Thigh

A series of quick, repetitive movements anywhere on the body will create an immediate burst of warm feelings that will stay with your partner for quite a while. On the thigh, you can spread warm sensation from knee to hip with a single long stroking movement. Be sure her thigh is well oiled because once you get the feeling of this stroke, it's fun to increase the speed. As long as you avoid slapping her and keep your contact even, there is no limit to how fast you can go. The same stroke works as well on the side of the back and on her lower leg.

Cup your hands around the top of your partner's leg so the thumb is opposite the other four fingers (as shown). Pull back all the way to the hip with first one hand, then the other.

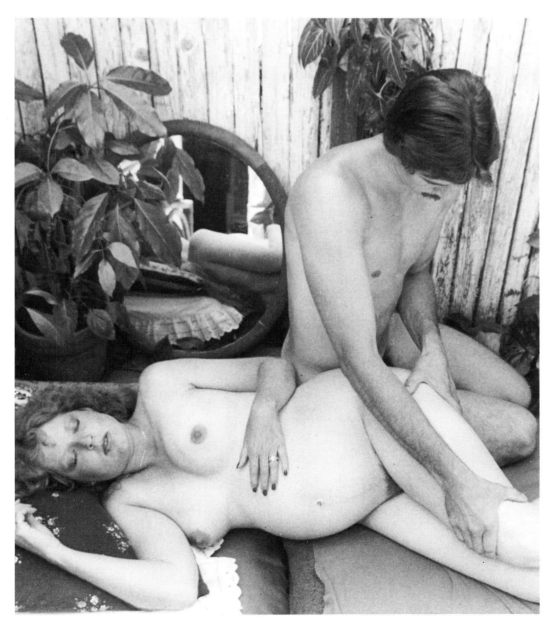

The Forearm Press

Usually, when masseurs want to relax the upper leg, they will concentrate on the four-part quadriceps muscle used in extending the knee joint. This powerful muscle runs from hip to knee and can be massaged without ever moving off the front of the thigh. Knead up and down it just a dozen times, and your partner will notice a difference the next day every time she climbs stairs.

From above and below, very powerful forces are focused on delicate structures inside the knee. We have all seen the kind of excruciating problems that develop when these forces get out of control. To help stabilize the whole joint, a fibrous band of muscle fascia runs down the side of the leg and presses against the knee joint. When your partner is on her back and the side of her leg is half-concealed, it's easy to ignore this band and bear down

twice as hard on the quadriceps. Unfortunately it's no easier to massage the side of the leg with your partner on her stomach since the other half of the leg disappears. But once she has rolled onto her side during the third trimester, you can easily reach the front, back, and side of the leg from a single spot. Be careful on the inside of the thigh where a rare surface artery makes anything but very light massage impossible.

Grasp one of your arms at the wrist to keep it steady and to distribute pressure evenly. Begin rotating your arm slowly just above your partner's knee, and press down while you turn. Then move up and down her thigh slowly as you continue rotating.

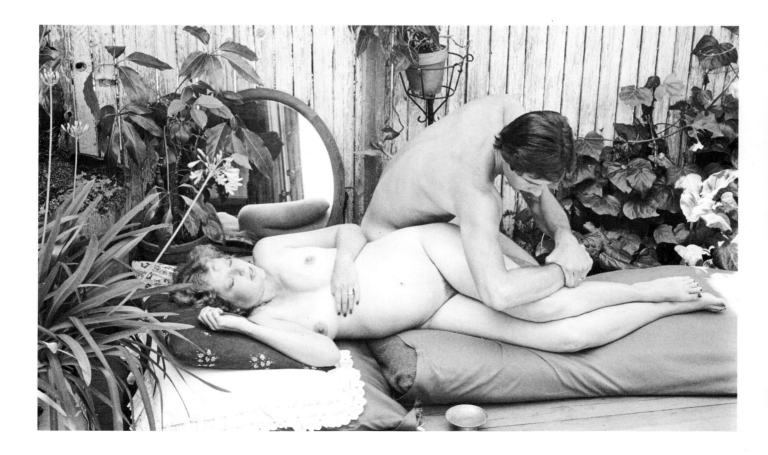

Once again, the right leg, where abdominal pressures can impede circulation as early as the second month, should receive extra attention. The forearm press will reach deep inside the leg to the large veins that run along the bone. Use it to stimulate blood and lymph circulation while you improve the tone of a major muscle group.

Be ready with plenty of oil because two large absorbent surfaces, your partner's thigh and your own forearm, are in constant contact. Oil your entire forearm before beginning, then, if tiny hairs knot up as you rotate, add extra oil. Try to avoid short scrubbing motions. This stroke permits a masseur with a taste for drama to stretch out and cover the whole thigh with a single uninterrupted circle.

The forearm press works well from either side of her body. Get comfortable before you begin. Be sure to put your oil nearby where you can get to it without having to move, and remember to have a soft towel handy. You will be oiling your entire forearm for this movement and may find that it's necessary to add oil before you're through. By simply changing the angle of your arm while you massage, you can move to the side of her leg and circle on the fibrous band that protects her knee. The forearm press can be extended to the back of her leg, but be sure to continue circling at the same rate. If your partner seems genuinely thrilled with what you've been doing, move down to the fleshy back of the lower leg. But no matter how enthusiastic she becomes, it's best to resist the temptation to press up onto her side and abdomen. Leave that part of the massage for after pregnancy, and concentrate, for now, on her hard-working legs.

Massaging the quadriceps is actually the first step in relaxing the body's most complex joint, the knee. Here, under the kneecap, amid a complex web of ligaments and tendons, muscles which spread out across the entire thigh are gathered.

The massive four-part quadriceps muscle spreads out across the thigh, then narrows to a single point at the knee.

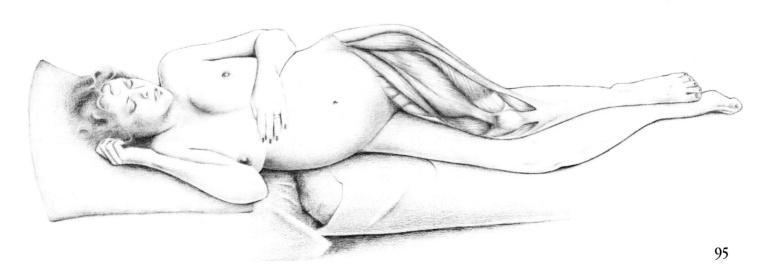

Knuckle Pressing

If the forearm press thrilled her, why not continue with more of the same? You're in the right position for several other movements that feel very good and will complement the softening-up process you just began. Large muscles, like the quadriceps, usually require a few different strokes to get them truly relaxed. Knuckle pressing allows you to bear down on a specific part of the muscle, a useful trick if your partner has been complaining about aches and pains in her legs.

Press down the thigh with the flat surface of your second knuckle, and steady your arm at the wrist with the other hand. You should be making contact with the second knuckle and the fleshy base of your palm. Circle slowly, moving your hand up and down her leg the same way you did in the forearm press. This stroke permits you to concentrate your pressure on a small area. Knuckle pressing is an ideal movement for fatigue and muscular pain.

When you want to relieve localized pain, sometimes nothing less than several *minutes* of circling on the same spot will do. This may mean repeating one movement hundreds of times, a prospect that makes new masseurs somewhat panicky. Will your carefully orchestrated massage rhythms suddenly collapse as fatigue takes its toll? Probably not. Climbing stairs, bicycling for just a few minutes, or even walking involves hundreds of repetitions of the same movement. You're using less practiced muscles in massage, but it's still something you should be able to handle. Remember: All that repetition may seem uninteresting, to everyone but your partner. The benefits of continually circling with knuckle pressing over one spot on a sore thigh can last for days. Muscles that have been cramped and oxygen-deprived are suddenly pumped full of nutrients; oxygen supplies are tripled, and fatigue-causing acids are drained from the tissues. Eventually you will begin to feel the whole area soften as what was once a source of constant irritation becomes just an unpleasant memory. The next day your partner may notice that the area you massaged actually feels *more* supple than other parts of the body. It is exactly this sort of amazing transformation that brings a woman back to massage throughout her pregnancy. The next time she feels a cramp beginning she'll come to you rather than reach for the pill bottle.

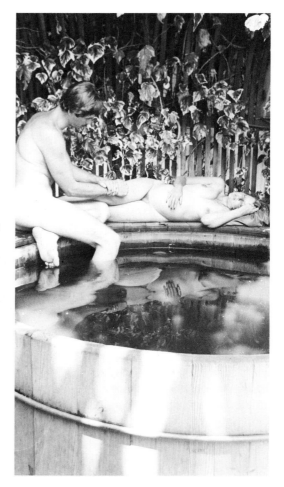

Knuckle pressing and the forearm press work well together. The two strokes can be blended by simply bending the wrist as you move onto the side of your partner's leg. Remember to circle, rather than scrub, with your hand and arm. Move down onto the side of her leg until your wrist makes contact with the thigh. Then, circling at the same speed, return to the top of her leg with the forearm press.

Spot Friction

If your partner is bothered by a nagging pain too deep to be reached by the forearm press or knuckle pressing, try some spot friction. It works even better here than on the back because it's easier for you to anchor on the rounded surface of her leg. Gather some flesh with your anchor hand, and push down gently. Move your friction hand into the area between thumb and forefinger, press down moderately hard, and circle on the underlying muscle tissue. While you circle, you may want to reposi-

tion your anchor hand occasionally as the gathered flesh begins to slip away.

Of course, your partner doesn't have to be hurting to enjoy friction. It feels particularly good around the joints, where the movement stimulates production of synovial fluid, an important lubricant.

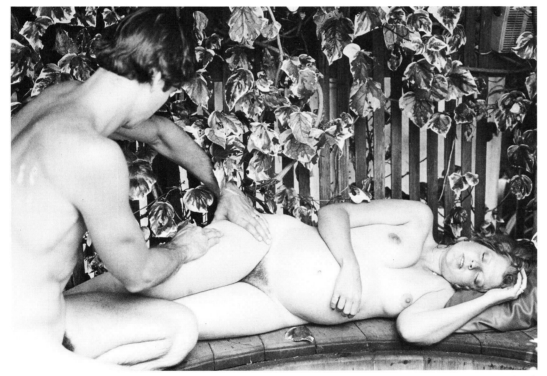

Full hand friction on the arm or leg can be anchored from the opposite side of the limb.

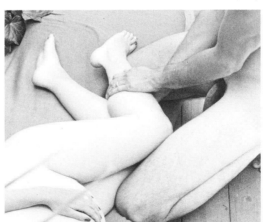

No extra oil is necessary during friction strokes. In a pinch, you can do spot friction to a sore joint or shoulder muscle without oil. Press down firmly enough so that your friction hand doesn't pull on the skin. Spot friction lets you feel things inside your partner's body.

97

Massaging the Mother and Child

The history of man for the first nine months preceding his birth would, probably, be far more interesting and contain events of greater moment than all the threescore and ten years that follow.

Samuel Taylor Coleridge

Before the third trimester has begun the baby exercises its limbs constantly, falls asleep when rocked, awakens when the motion stops, becomes agitated when the mother is angry and relaxes as she calms down. No greater intimacy is possible between two human beings.

Please the mother, and you benefit her child.

We live in a century in which everything secret eventually manages to get photographed and exhibited somewhere. Even the pharaohs, who desperately sought peace and privacy, have been carefully removed from the centers of their pyramids to be routinely photographed by bored schoolchildren in the British Museum. Once the most thoroughly dead people on earth had been exhibited, most scientists were content to focus on more modest animal kingdom members. Still, a single unlikely frontier remained, and it was left to a team of Swedish researchers armed with a persistent little camera to peer finally into the womb itself, illuminating (with high-intensity flash) the only period in the life or death of man that had never been photographed. Unfortunately the fetus was hardly more cooperative than the pharaohs, and inside the womb, the researchers were thoroughly ignored by a Buddha-like creature floating peacefully near the mother's heart but already living a separate life. This discovery brought considerable speculation on the precise relationship between a fetus and the world outside a mother's body. Does the fetus "see" anything? Can it hear music or somehow understand certain words? Beyond these purely mechanical questions is a more esoteric one that's seldom asked: Does the fetus have a secret life which every adult has completely forgotten?

As an individual a fetus has experiences that are sometimes shared with the mother but that can also be private and utterly mysterious. The tactile sense, the primary sense of single-celled animals, provides nearly the whole connection between a fetus and the outside world. Practically everything that is experienced for the first nine months of human life is simply felt. This is the most perfectly sensual period in any person's life, and you can contribute to it, for a few minutes, when you massage a pregnant woman's abdomen.

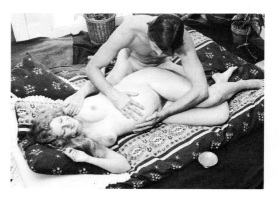

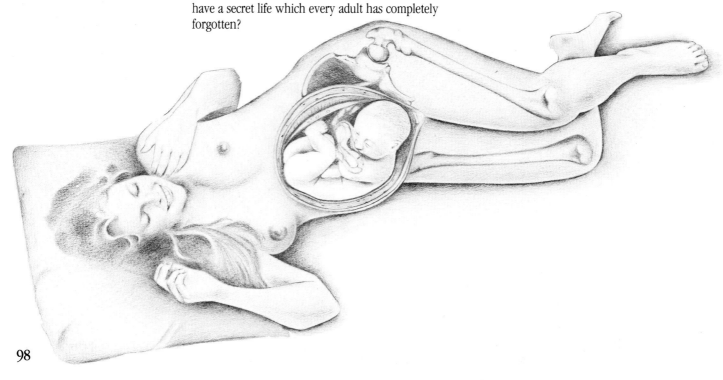

Kneading the Abdomen

You can use either fingertip or full-hand kneading strokes across the abdomen. Since your massage here will definitely be felt by the fetus as well as by the mother, it's a good idea to introduce slowly the idea of direct abdominal contact. Carefully lift the side of her abdomen with the full surface of one hand, and simply hold her for a few moments. Whether or not you can actually feel the baby, a gentle pause allows the mother and baby to get comfortable with the new feeling. It will also permit you to test the skin tension across the mother's belly, which varies from week to week, even from day to day. If it seems very tight, concentrate on full-hand kneading, and avoid the fingertip variation, which really works better with looser skin.

This is another one of the strokes for which feedback is invaluable. Tell your partner this before you begin the massage so she will be ready to participate. Kneading the abdomen is a happy stroke because it brings the three of you very close together. Some of the loveliest smiles you see during massage come after this movement.

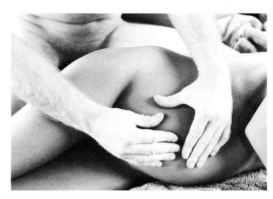

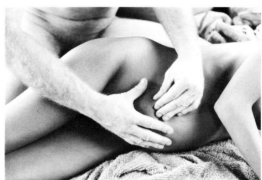

Get comfortable so you don't have to rearrange yourself. Cup your hands to fit the curve of your partner's belly. In late pregnancy kneading becomes a surface stroke that concentrates on the skin. Avoid any kind of deep pressure. Try the stroke a few times and proceed according to your partner's wishes. If you get to the belly after a lot of massage and she's too relaxed to talk stay with light contact and full hand kneading.

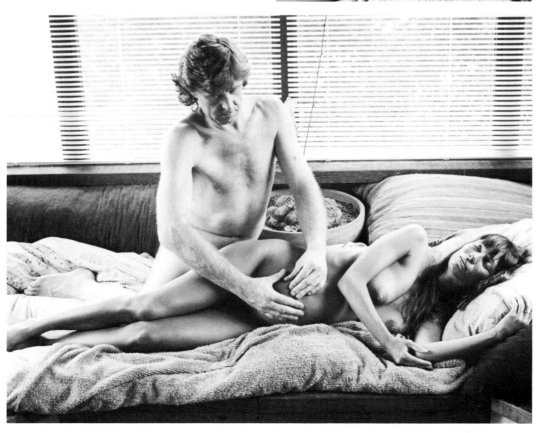

Move up and back across the abdomen from breastbone to the bottom of the belly until you've covered the whole area. At the very top of this stroke, you can lean back a bit and knead the whole side of her body from armpit to knee. Be sure to lift her top arm with both hands and bring it forward before you do this.

99

Light Belly Friction

If your partner enjoyed having her belly kneaded enough to ask for more massage in that area, try some gentle broad-handed belly friction. Here again, it's important to be sure you're well balanced and comfortable before you begin.

Like fingertip kneading, very light, sensitive belly friction will almost always please a pregnant woman, and once you have begun, your partner will probably want the feeling to continue for a while. Even a light friction stroke can be fatiguing if it's extended for a long time. If you feel tired, keep

contact with her body and allow yourself a brief rest. When your partner reclines with her legs forward, light belly friction becomes easier by resting the elbow of your anchor hand lightly on her thigh, just above the knee.

Belly friction travels particularly well. You're beginning from a point near the center of her body and will have no trouble reaching down onto her thigh or up the side of her body as far as the shoulder. If you decide to do this, use extra pressure as the stroke blends with other friction movements over heavily muscled parts of her body, like the thighs and upper arms. Pay special attention to the massive hip joint, where increased pressure will allow you to reach deep inside.

Slide one hand under her stomach just far enough to anchor the stroke, and press the other hand onto her belly. Keep your fingers together, and begin rotating the friction hand in small circles. Use light pressure on this stroke, and be prepared to stop and go on to another movement if she becomes uncomfortable.

Use less pressure on the inside of the arm and thigh during kneading and stroking movements. This simple precaution is especially important when you are massaging towards the heart—against the flow of surface arteries.

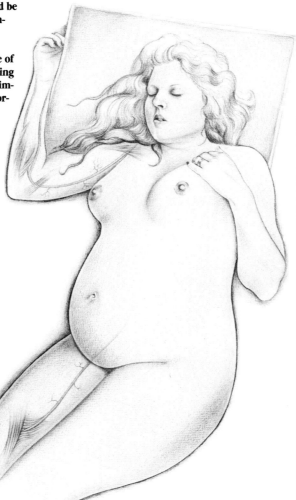

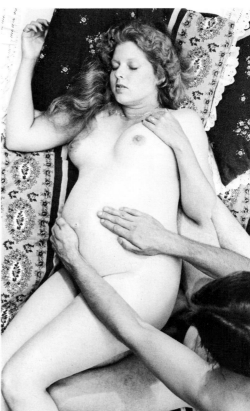

The Full Body Sweep

This incomparable movement spreads pleasure to the whole length of your partner's body and should be included whenever you do more than a few minutes of massage. Even if you massage only her back and abdomen, the full body sweep will leave a woman with the feeling that you've given some attention to every part of her body.

Begin by laying your hands flat on your partner's hip, thumbs touching and fingers parallel. Cup your fingers and palms so your hands will mold themselves to the changing shape of her body as you stroke. Press outward from the hip, moving one hand down toward the feet and the other up toward the shoulder. Spread your arms as far as you can comfortably, and stop. Hold the extended position for a few moments before reversing the stroke and returning to her hip. Unlike back massage, the return movement here is not superficial and requires pressures which are just as strong as the beginning stroke. What your partner *feels* is a single lush sweep up and down the whole side of her body. Repeat the full body sweep at least three times, but don't stop then if she's grinning and sighing.

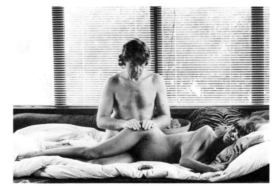

The most luxurious full body sweep is the most generous stroke in massage. Expect to add more oil, especially if you're planning on lots of repetition. Get comfortable near the center of your partner's body and stroke out as far as you can without unbalancing yourself. Cup your hands to fit the changing shape of her body and maintain a consistent rhythm out to the far ends of the movement.

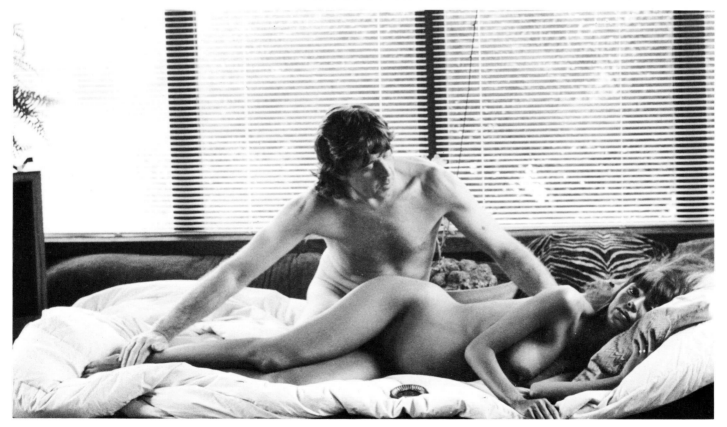

Brushing the Body: A Sensation Transfer

Brushing is an exception to two of the basic rules of massage: You do it with only your fingertips, and you keep your fingers spread wide apart. Begin by sitting near the midpoint of your partner's body where you can easily reach her shoulders. Brushing involves repetitive short movements that descend gradually from the shoulders to the feet. As the stroke moves down your partner's body, you may want to move with it if you find reaching toward the feet difficult. Usually brushing strokes are about a foot long, but it's fun to vary the length and, occa-

sionally, the speed of individual movements. Try beginning with a series of very short downward strokes, slowly lengthening them until each sequence covers half a leg or more. The sides of the legs are particularly sensitive, and if your reach is long enough, you can eventually brush the whole leg in one long, sweeping motion that begins at the hip and ends on the toes. And the toes, often neglected by even the most experienced masseurs, are a good place to end your brushing movement especially if you plan to have your partner turn over so you can then massage the other leg. As your fingers glide down the lower leg, think about ending your final stroke on her toes. Brush across the bottom of her foot until the fingers of one hand meet the tips of her toes. Hold that contact for a full minute, and as you break it gradually, press your free hand onto her other leg. This gentle transition allows your partner to feel the massage being moved from one part of her body to another.

When brushing the toes you may discover that your partner is ticklish. She may still be nervous about being massaged or just overly sensitive on a small part of her body. To avoid interrupting the massage it's best to respect her sensitivity and go on to another part of the body.

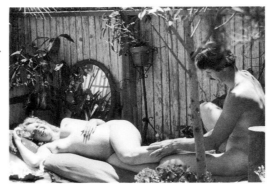

Make contact with the sides of your partner's fingers at the end of arm brushing. The sides are far more sensitive than the tops and bottoms.

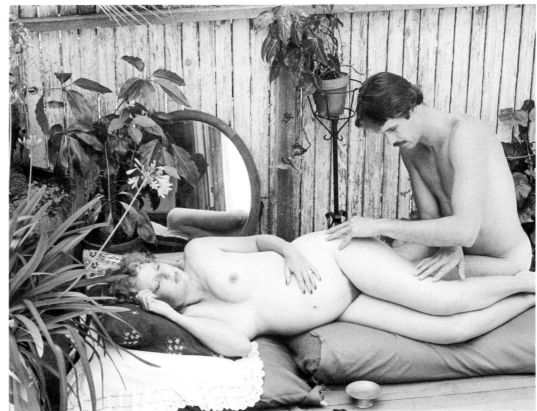

It isn't necessary to adapt to any radical new situations when you massage your partner's head and neck in the side lying position. Just refer to the complete head massage section in early pregnancy (see page 69). The neck is flexible enough to give you plenty of room to work, even though her face will be turned to one side. You do need to watch the position of her shoulders. If they're tilted forward, her head will roll all the way to one side. With the shoulders vertical or even tilted back slightly, you will have a much easier time massaging her head. If she's in the shoulder forward position when you begin, simply ask her to roll back or, even better, help her make the change while you ask. Whenever your partner needs to move, it's always better for you to get involved in repositioning limbs rather than sit passively and issue instructions which can be easily misunderstood.

Lift your partner's arm above and below the elbow, and place it along her side so the forearm is resting just above her belly. If you want to bring her arm back even farther, the elbow will drop behind her side, and you should be sure to support it with a pillow. Once you've positioned her arm, it's time to think about moving her whole upper body to the side. Gently push back on the front of her shoulder with one hand while supporting the back of the shoulder with the other. Move her until the chin comes up and she reaches a comfortable position. You may want to put a small pillow behind her shoulder blade for extra support. Use the edge of one hand to hold the down side of her face while you massage her neck.

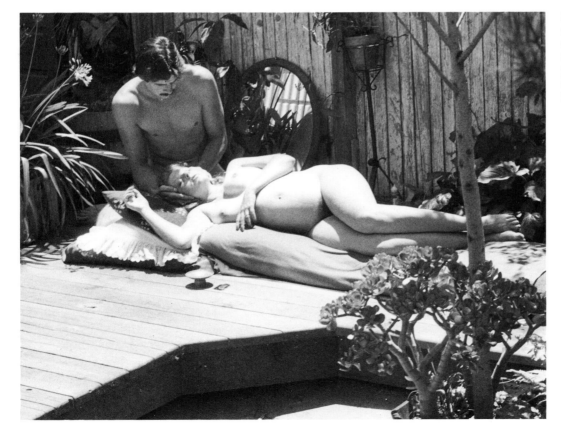

Be sure your knees are adequately cushioned and leave yourself enough room to lean back occasionally. Put the oil next to one of your partner's shoulders. You won't need much if you've been massaging another part of her body.

A COMPLETE
BACK MASSAGE

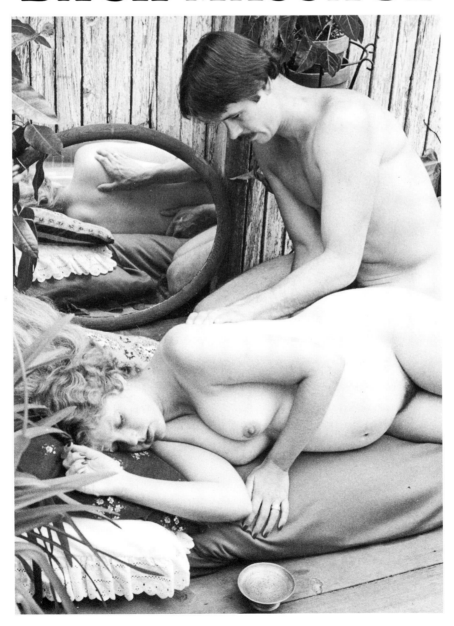

The Baby and the Lower Back

During pregnancy all the major bones of the lower back will move to accommodate the expanding uterus. The two small lower ribs, the only ones not connected to the sternum on the front of the body, change position easily. The spine and pelvis, however, contain some of the largest bone structures in the body, and when they are moved, muscles, tendons, and ligaments are stretched. We usually think of the skeleton as an anchoring point for all the muscles of the body, but there are muscles which actually support a part of the skeletal system. Long

muscles that run parallel to the spine stabilize the vertebrae and hold them erect. Several major leg and torso muscles which are supported by the skeleton in the usual way are stretched when large pelvic bones begin to shift. Muscles move the body by contracting and must then return to a completely relaxed state to gather energy. If a muscle is not permitted to relax or is stretched too far, it's likely to cramp.

A thorough back massage should include large muscles from other parts of the body that tie into the back and exert powerful forces on the spine. Some begin near the spine and provide support for parts of the limbs and torso, while others influence the back from a remote position. A wide band of muscles called the external obliques begins on the back and wraps around a woman's belly to support it. These muscles are used whenever the back is flexed as a woman moves from a sitting to a standing position. Just beneath the external obliques, running vertically across the belly, are the powerful rectus abdominis muscles, which give support to the womb and help lift the torso whenever she sits up from a reclining

Every part of the lower back skeleton will change position during pregnancy.

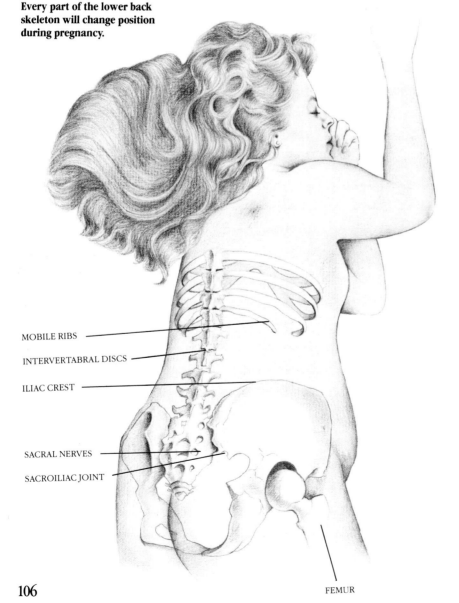

MOBILE RIBS

INTERVERTABRAL DISCS

ILIAC CREST

SACRAL NERVES

SACROILIAC JOINT

FEMUR

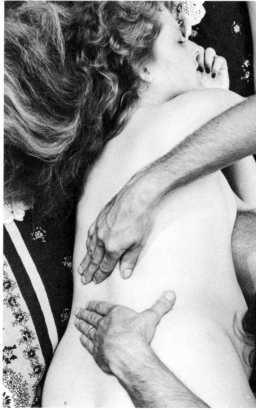

position. Muscles of the abdomen and lumbar back work together to carry the fetus *and* support the mother-to-be. They are used nearly every time a woman moves and are put under increasing strain as the womb expands.

Almost all the muscles, ligaments, and tendons of the lower back are stretched beyond their normal limits during pregnancy. A small relatively obscure ligament, called the uterosacral, that anchors the bottom of the uterus to the lower spine is suddenly required to support a large part of the weight of a developing fetus. As it's stretched by the growing womb, there is a constant danger that this ligament will become the source of a painful and frustrating internal sprain. Unfortunately the uterosacral ligament is too deep within the abdomen to be massaged directly, but you can considerably reduce the chance of its being sprained or torn by relaxing the surrounding tissues.

Remember, severely cramped lumbar muscles can twist the spine, pinch nerves, and send shooting pains down the legs. If nothing is done and the problem recurs, the intervertebral disks may be damaged.

Too many women endure that kind of punishment when regular back massage could have been used to keep the lower-back muscles toned and supple while they are stretched into a new shape.

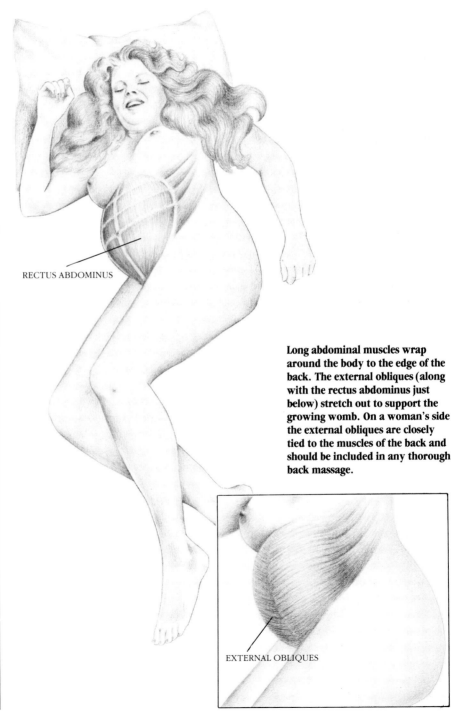

RECTUS ABDOMINUS

Long abdominal muscles wrap around the body to the edge of the back. The external obliques (along with the rectus abdominus just below) stretch out to support the growing womb. On a woman's side the external obliques are closely tied to the muscles of the back and should be included in any thorough back massage.

EXTERNAL OBLIQUES

6

Breasts, Back, and Belly

As breasts and belly grow during pregnancy, most of the extra body weight is carried by the muscles of the lower back. These muscles support the torso and keep the spine in position. When a woman begins to gain weight rapidly, she is likely to experience persistent fatigue in the lower back, even though she exercises. If her weight gain is great, major muscles of the lower back may begin to weaken just when extra strength is necessary. This becomes a particularly dangerous situation when the erector muscles that support the spine are weak-

ened. A slight change in the spine's normal curve can have serious consequences for a pregnant woman, whose posture determines the way her baby will be carried.

Extra weight, particularly in the abdominal region, can put so much pressure on the lower spine that a condition known as lordosis, or swayback, develops. A slight forward shift in the position of the lower spine pushes the abdomen forward and forces the upper torso far enough back to unbalance her entire body. As lower-back muscles become overfatigued

A minor shift in the position of a pregnant woman's back and abdomen moves the center of balance all the way off the back of her body.

Postural changes (see opposite) eventually affect the carrying angle of the fetus. As the carrying angle becomes more awkward new stresses are put on the back creating a vicious circle of accumulating tension.

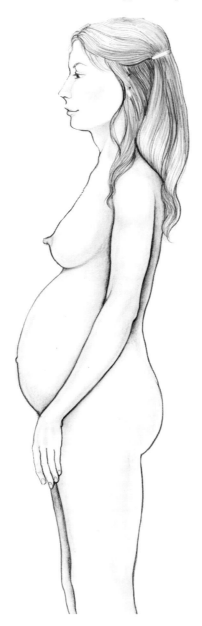
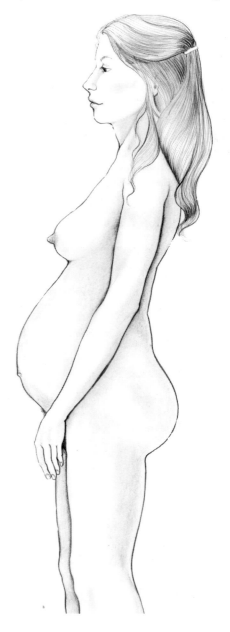

and weaken, connective tissue around the spine begins to shorten. Finally, the abdomen is thrust forward, pulling the spine with it, and the pattern of pressure distribution on the vertebrae begins to change. Normally the task of supporting and carrying the body is distributed in equal parts to the whole spine. When great pressures begin to build in the lumbar region, your partner is headed for painful nerve and disk problems.

As the fetus develops and the abdomen and breasts begin swelling, swayback becomes difficult to recognize. It's easy to attribute any new body profile to the changes every woman expects during pregnancy, but if she's complaining of lower-back pain, it's useful to look carefully at her side standing posture. A relatively minor shift in the position of her lower back and abdomen throws the center of balance all the way off the back of her body. Then, as the abdomen and breasts continue to grow and more weight must be supported, the swayback becomes a bit more pronounced. When tremendous pressures begin building on lower-back vertebrae and nerves, the entire torso may tighten from hips to shoulders.

Eventually her condition becomes so tense that a single sudden, unusual motion (like a cough) is enough to produce spasm and excruciating pain.

Fortunately the human body is plastic enough to recover from all sorts of disfiguring injuries, and you can correct a postural problem with regular exercise and massage.

THE CENTER OF BALANCE   THE CENTER OF BALANCE

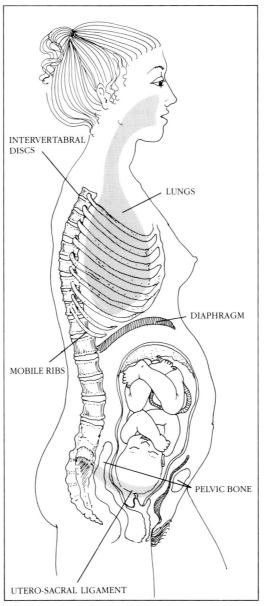

INTERVERTABRAL DISCS

LUNGS

DIAPHRAGM

MOBILE RIBS

PELVIC BONE

UTERO-SACRAL LIGAMENT

Pressure from the growing womb restricts the diaphragm and pushes up on the two "mobile" lowest ribs. The uterosacral ligament pulls forward on the lower spine compressing the intervertebral disks. By the time major pubic bones begin to shift the stomach and intestines have been reshaped.

Massaging a Sore Back

. . . in the midst of an attack so severe that she could not get out of bed, [she] phoned and begged that a prescription for a narcotic be phoned to her druggist. Instead, I got to her as soon as possible and listened to her report that she had not slept for two nights and now could hardly even roll from one side of the bed to the other. Examination revealed severe muscle spasm, and the first measure I used was massage. Within just a few minutes she was able to get out of bed and get to the bathroom.

Lawrence W. Friedmann, M.D.

Anyone who has suffered from intense fatigue, sudden cramping, or muscle spasm knows that there are several kinds of back pain. Low-level pain that makes bending from the waist difficult is often rationalized or ignored during pregnancy. Women who have not been massaged may remind you that they are constantly adjusting to new aches and pains; one more in the lower back seems like a minor annoyance. Should she simply avoid lifting anything heavy and remind friends that pregnancy has given her a (temporary) bad back? Perhaps she should focus on other things and try to forget about low-level back pain. That kind of thinking often leads to the other kind of back pain, which cannot be ignored or rationalized because it's so intense.

There is no reason why a pregnant woman should endure pain that can easily be vanquished by regular massage. Low-level pain and persistent stiffness are useful warnings of worse things to come; it's best to respond with fluid release massage instead of apathy or panic. With plenty of repetition, the strokes in this section can make a major difference after a single massage. Ask your partner to sample them before she reaches for a bottle of pain pills. After a few minutes, while oxygen and nutrients are pumped into congested tissues, you will feel muscles begin to soften under your hands as her back relaxes.

If back pain is intense and includes shooting pains down the legs, your partner may have disk problems, and it's best to get the advice of an orthopedic doctor before beginning with massage. Hopefully, the doctor will find no structural problems. Simple sprains and cramps can be just as painful as the dreaded slipped disk without having lasting effects.

The usual response to intense lower-back pain is rest in a firm bed followed by a program of back-strengthening exercises. Unfortunately this well-meaning plan can create unexpected problems for a masseur and his pregnant partner. Almost everyone manages to observe part one of the plan because, usually, after a lower-back muscle spasm there is no other choice. However, the rest period, with its enforced inactivity, can encourage a pregnant woman to make unrealistic resolutions that will eventually create more problems. When her back hurts so much she can't put on her own shoes, it's comforting to plan the most ambitious exercise programs. But if she's never practiced yoga, calisthen-ics, or aerobic dancing, the first painless day after a back injury is a dangerous time to begin.

Under the best conditions people recover from back problems by degree. Rushing things, particularly during pregnancy, is almost always the road to painful relapse and more colorful exercise fantasies.

Massage may be so therapeutic that a woman will try too much too soon. Ten minutes spent kneading and stroking aching lower-back muscles will often result in a feeling of total relief. This time, however, the feeling may be deceptive. Inside the back a swollen disk or muscle may still be pressing hard on a nerve. Simply rising too fast from the massage surface can put the muscles back into spasm even though you succeeded in relaxing them temporarily. After you're through stroking, it's a good idea to help your partner rise from the massage surface. Do this by having her hold onto the back of your neck while the two of you sit up slowly. If she has been experiencing intense back pain, it's helpful to warn her not to overexercise the moment she feels relief.

Any competent obstetrician can recommend simple but effective exercises for the back. Well-massaged women may want to go farther and consider the thiry-minute-a-day exercise program described in a wonderful little book called *Freedom from Backaches,* by Lawrence W. Friedmann, M.D., and Lawrence Galton (New York: Simon & Schuster, 1973), which delivers exactly what it promises.

Once the back actually does begin to mend after regular massage and selected exercise, your partner sometimes faces a new set of problems. Exercises that were refreshing a week ago may now seem dull and terribly remedial. Instead of solving your partner's back problems, they manage only to remind her of them. It's easy to remember sickness and be repelled by it, but the specific sensation of pain can never be recalled. You may have to remind your partner that back massage works best if it's supplemented by a carefully planned exercise program. You can relax and tone her muscles with massage, but to remain strong, they must be exercised.

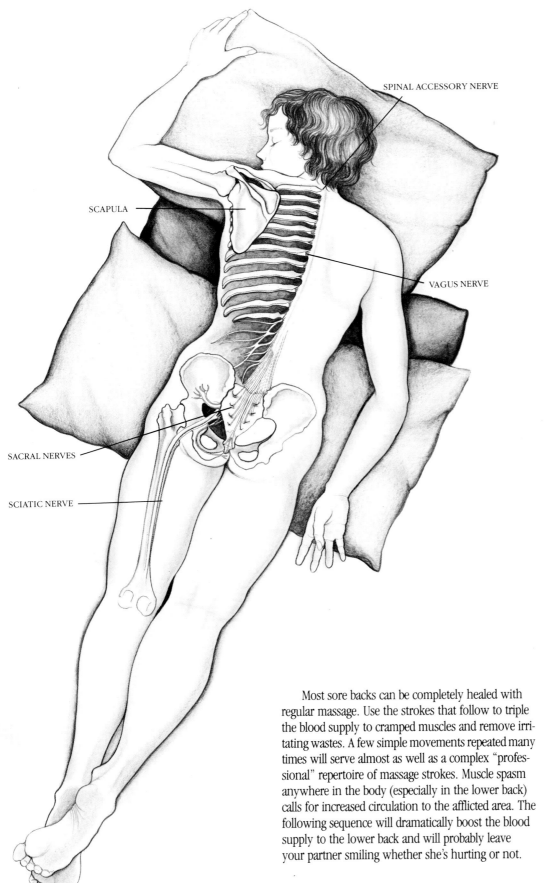

SPINAL ACCESSORY NERVE

SCAPULA

VAGUS NERVE

SACRAL NERVES

SCIATIC NERVE

The primary nerves of the back run parallel to the bottom of the ribs. Major nerves of the legs run through spaces between the pelvic bones.

The same strokes that help muscles stretch into new positions while the bones move will bring relief in cases of spasm. Here you must make use of the fluid release effect. Be patient, and be ready for plenty of repetition. The specific techniques you will need to help her relax (so that exercise can begin) are included in the section that follows.

If your partner raises an arm above her head (as shown) the scapula is elevated. This makes upper back massage more difficult.

Most sore backs can be completely healed with regular massage. Use the strokes that follow to triple the blood supply to cramped muscles and remove irritating wastes. A few simple movements repeated many times will serve almost as well as a complex "professional" repertoire of massage strokes. Muscle spasm anywhere in the body (especially in the lower back) calls for increased circulation to the afflicted area. The following sequence will dramatically boost the blood supply to the lower back and will probably leave your partner smiling whether she's hurting or not.

111

6

Back Circulation

Back circulation, normally a powerful two-handed stroke, can be adapted for use in late pregnancy without losing much of its deep-penetrating effect. The idea is to anchor your partner's torso with one hand while you massage with the other. Do this by sliding your anchor hand under her waist (as shown) and lifting up slightly with your fingertips. Your anchor hand should give her just enough support to keep the torso from rolling forward when stroking begins. You'll be massaging along the side of her spine from the hip to the top of the shoulder.

A little feedback from your partner will help you locate exactly the right spot to press—she's going to be very sensitive around the sides of her belly.

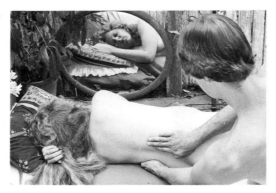

an inch away above the raised spinal muscles.

Once both hands are in position, you're ready to begin one of the most satisfying strokes in massage. Your partner may ask you to repeat this movement over and over again; get it right, and you will be able to give her exactly what she wants. Most women enjoy fairly high pressure on the rows of raised muscles that run parallel to the spine. Concentrate pressure on the lower back with the base of the palm, but again, remember to avoid direct pressure on the spine.

Perhaps because it covers so much territory, there's a temptation to rush this movement and skip part of the shoulder or even to break contact at the bottom of the back. To avoid these common mistakes, concentrate on keeping your pressure even, and make the entire stroke a single uninterrupted sweep up the back and down the side. Get it just right and you may be rewarded by the peaceful sigh or gentle inward smile so familiar to experienced masseurs.

It's important to keep your whole hand, right up to the fingertips, in contact with your partner's back. As you approach her shoulder, transfer the pressure from the base of the palm to your fingers. Bend your fingers across the collarbone until your whole hand fits, half-moon-style, over her shoulder. At this point, as you move out from the neck to the side of her back with your fingers curled over her shoulder, pressures should be evenly distributed from the heel of your hand to the fingertips. The return part of the stroke moves down the side of her back, with your fingers wrapping almost far enough around to touch her belly. Pressure on the return should be light to moderate. At the base of her back you will be ready to turn again and return to your original position.

Begin by placing your free hand on the side of your partner's hip at the base of the back. Keep your fingers together, and press into the muscles of her back. It's important to be careful not to press hard on the spine at any time when you're doing massage. Any contact you make with it should be light and superficial. You may want to tuck the tip of your thumb under your forefinger (as shown) to be sure that you don't dig into her spine with your thumb as you move up the back. The thumb side of your hand should be parallel to the spine and about

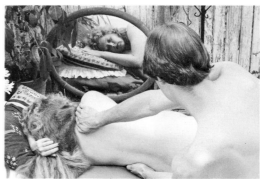

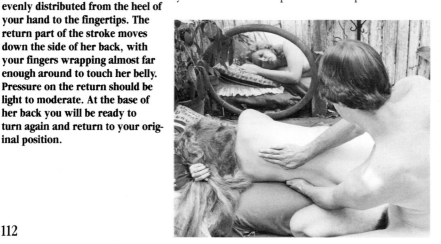

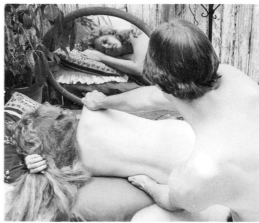

If your partner seems blissful after a few minutes of circulation strokes, she probably will appreciate more massage over the same area. Here is a movement you can use to provide a new and very refreshing sensation on the long muscles that run parallel to the spine. You've already started to relax them. Why not continue with something very soothing? Effective thumb stroking requires lots of repetition on both sides of the spine. Since you won't be using as much pressure as you did during circulation stroking, your partner isn't likely to roll forward, and anchoring is not necessary. As extra insurance, you can arrange her arms in one of the positions shown. She won't need to actually do anything, but the position of her hand and elbows will provide the extra measure of support you will need to keep her steady. This is another long stroke, and positioning yourself well at the beginning will help you remain comfortable while reaching both ends of the back.

Be sure that four fingers of each hand stay in contact with the back while your thumbs are massaging. As long as you remember to lift your hands

one at a time, you won't risk abandoning your partner altogether. Use moderate pressures; you should be able to see your thumbs depress the flesh a bit. Remember to stay off the spine itself; the muscles you want are usually visible all the way from neck to hip. Begin with short, alternating strokes up at the neck, and work your way down to the lower back slowly. Again, repetition will mean more to your partner than a quick trip down the back. If she's tense, keep at it until you begin to feel sections of the muscles soften as they are

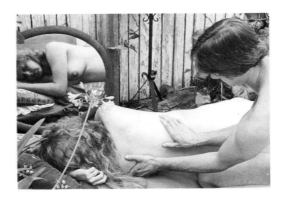 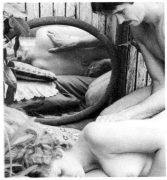

massaged. Down on the hips you can easily vary the length of your strokes. It's always fun to cover the whole back with one stroke for a while and then go back to shorter strokes like the ones you used in the beginning.

Open your hands, and lay them on the top of your partner's back with each of your thumbs flat against the long muscles that run parallel to her spine. Hold your thumbs in that position, and stroke down along the spine, lifting one hand and then the other to return to the top position. Begin by stroking a quarter of the way down the back before lifting your hand; you'll have a chance to modify the stroke later.

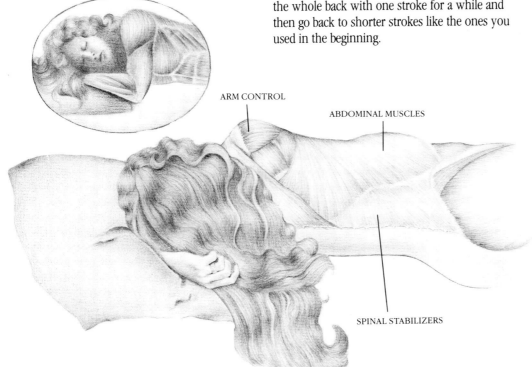

ARM CONTROL

ABDOMINAL MUSCLES

SPINAL STABILIZERS

To fully relax the arms or the abdomen you must massage the muscles of the back.

Pressing the Spinal Muscles

Inside the spine, thirty-one pairs of bundled nerves connect the brain with every part of the body. The spine is actually an extension of the lower brain, and like the brain, it is entirely anesthetic. Nothing is felt inside when you work around the spine, but the usual internal changes do take place: The nerves are stimulated, internal circulation increases, and the muscle tone of surrounding tissues begins to improve. Apart from a tiny spot at the base of the skull, massaging around the spine is about as close as you can get to massaging the brain itself.

Light to moderate pressures work best, but of course, every woman will have her perference. If you're unsure exactly how much pressure to use, use less. All the pressure is focused on the oiled tips of your fingers, which press into the surrounding muscles as you move up the spine. Go all the way to the tops of the shoulders; then return to the hips with a light brushing stroke. Be sure to repeat the movement a few more times. During this stroke you are massaging nerve beginnings that supply nearly every part of your partner's body. After a

Spread the fingers of one hand so the spine can pass between them, arching your hand slightly. Grasp your contact arm just above the wrist, and press down gently onto the muscle that runs parallel to your partner's spine. Let the soft, fleshy base of your palm ride lightly over her spine. Be sure to get some feedback from your partner when you're learning this movement.

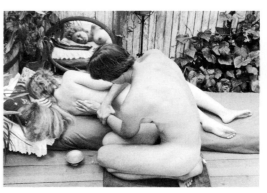

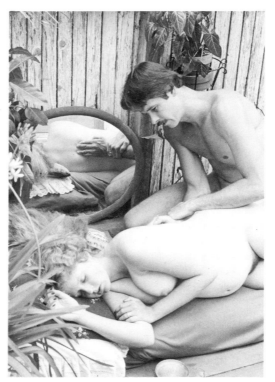

third or fourth repetition tensed intervertebral ligaments begin to relax, and your partner experiences a gentle ascending wave of pleasure that spreads through the whole torso.

Two-Handed Back Compression

Begin on the lower back with your hands opposed, and mold your fingers to the shape of your partner's side. It's particularly important during this movement to remember to maintain contact all the way from the base of your hand to the tips of your fingers. With almost any variation of the side lying position, your partner is likely to roll when you press forward with both hands at once. The trick is to press up with the fingers of your lower hand for extra support just enough to keep your partner from rolling when you push forward with the base of your hands.

After an initial pass up and down the back, you'll begin to feel exactly where you need to go with your lower hand to give extra support. At that point this stroke, like every other massage movement, becomes effortless, and you can settle down to enjoy giving your partner as much pleasure as possible.

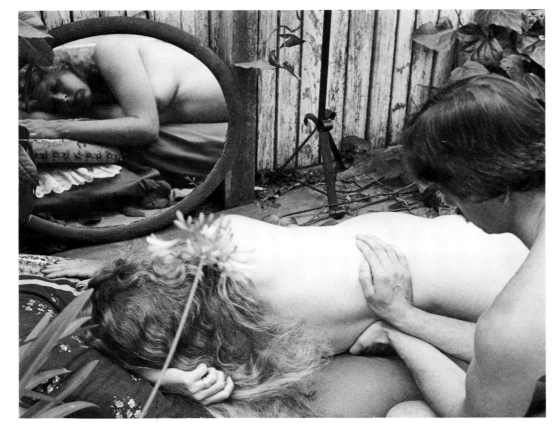

Move up her back one hand width at a time, pressing at least twice each time you stop. As you approach the top of the back, steady the movement by cupping the side of her shoulder with your anchor hand.

Spot Friction

The most basic sort of feedback you will need from a pregnant woman are directions on where to massage when she feels pain. Follow them, and when you reach the tender spot, use both hands to deliver a friction stroke that doesn't wander. Before you actually begin massaging, look carefully at the painful area to be sure there are no visible bruises, abrasions, or cuts. Sore muscles will usually respond to friction, particularly if you begin from a nearby point and approach the distressed area slowly. That way the massage sensation can grow until it gradually replaces the pain.

Every mammal instinctively understands that a painful spot must be rubbed. Your partner will let you know when you've found the right spot, and then nothing more needs to be said. Whether she's hurting or not, a woman will appreciate spot friction strokes that concentrate the effects of massage deep within her body.

Press down on your contact hand until it sinks into the flesh, and then push down from above with your anchor hand to gather even more flesh. Move in slowly until the painful spot is right between your thumb and forefinger. If the spot is very small, bring your fingers together to concentrate the stroke. The flat fingertips of your friction hand can then press into soft flesh and circle slowly. You'll need to reposition your anchor hand occasionally as the flesh continues to slip away under your fingers. Keep pressing it down from above without breaking the friction rhythm.

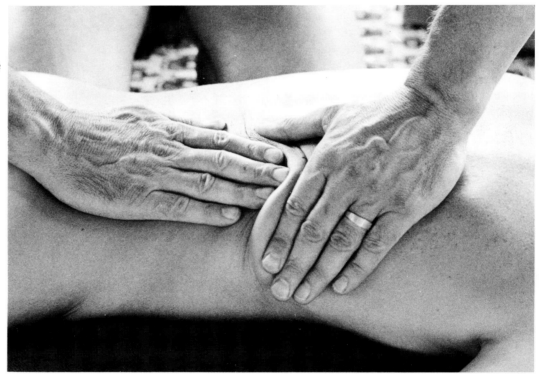

A common friction movement mistake: People fit together naturally during massage. No movement should feel awkward.

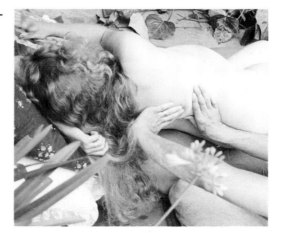

Shoulder Rotation

Almost every woman will enjoy the luxurious feeling of having a part of her body float through the air while she does nothing at all. Antigravity effects are one of the basic amenities in massage and really should not be missed. With a little effort from you, and none whatsoever from your partner, feet, hands, arms, fingers, toes, legs, assorted joints, and even the head will rotate freely. After a while a new masseur begins to discover interesting ways to levitate the most unlikely parts of a woman's body.

During a back massage your hands are never far from the spine, which is conveniently divided into thirty-four vertebrae, most of which move. This would be the ideal place to begin your levitation experiments were it not for the fact that the vertebrae are tied together and tend to move each other. Unless you want to start twisting the body into perilous shapes, the range of movement available to an individual vertebra during massage is very limited. The joints that move most effectively are not on the spine at all but rather up at the top of the back under the shoulder blade. While the vertebrae are tied together in a long flexible cord, these massive joints will rotate independently of the surrounding tissues.

Many people are greatly surprised the first time this movement is experienced. They simply never realized their shoulders could be lifted and rotated while the rest of the body remained still. This part of the massage actually becomes easier as a pregnancy develops and your partner turns on her side to stay comfortable.

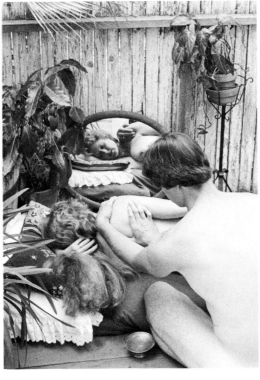

Wrap one hand over her shoulder just far enough to grasp the front of her arm. As you pull back gently, the massive shoulder joint will appear and become increasingly well defined. Your other hand will fit right over it, with the fingertips pressed over the bulge and the thumb tucked into the depression near her spine. Now simply push your hands together, and begin turning the whole joint. The upper arm will move a bit, but the rest of her body should remain perfectly still while you test the range of movement that's comfortable for her. When you feel resistance, back off slightly, and rotate the whole joint in a smooth circle just inside the point of resistance.

As the joint turns, try moving your thumb from the center of her back to the side (as shown). This extra measure of support will help your partner feel comfortable and cared for while she's relaxing.

117

"…at a child's birth, if a mother could ask a fairy godmother
to endow it with the most useful gift, that gift would be curiosity."

Eleanor Roosevelt

THE BIRTH

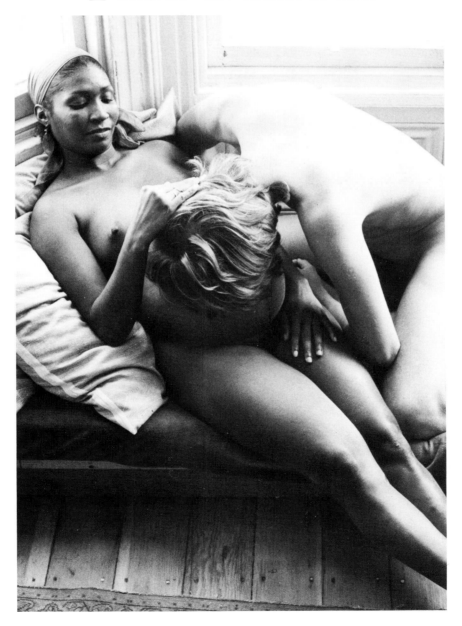

7

What To Do While You're Waiting for the Baby

. . . the individual, in his growth from meeting of sperm and ovum at conception, lives out, in fetus, the growth and evolution of his tribe: . . . first he is an amoeba, then a colonial organism, then an invertebrate, then a lancet, then a fish, until at last he is a mammal and a human.

Michael McClure

The precise way a woman will feel during labor is difficult to predict—the more so if this is her first baby. Some women will adore you for massaging them between contractions while others prefer not to be touched. Hopefully, you've learned massage technique by now (the birth is not a good time to begin practicing) and will be ready to help if you're called upon to do so. If you're not called upon right away, you may have to be content with pacing around in a small room and becoming furiously worried. Most of my ancestors were born while their fathers performed this ancient dance, and most likely yours were, too.

Excessive stress can turn an easy labor into a terrible ordeal. The degrading effects of stress on every body system are particularly worrisome during labor when overtensed abdominal muscles can delay a birth for hours. Anything you can do to relax a woman and reduce tension levels in her muscles will help her through this difficult period. There are two important ways a woman can become overstressed and very tense during labor: She can react to physical changes inside her body or

to disturbances in the birthing environment. Fortunately massage can help reduce tension from both sources.

Every woman must find a good way to relax between contractions during labor. If she decides on massage—and many women who have been massaged throughout pregnancy do—you will be ready with a complete repertoire of movements to dissolve muscular tension. You've worked with her for months, watched her change, and become familiar with her body. You know what to do for headaches and cramps; many times you've managed to substitute peace for panic. You know how to use your hands to feel for tension all over her body. You remain confident and relaxed no matter what position she must assume in order to get comfortable; you've practiced with all of them. Reaching for the oil bottle and a nearby towel, you hear her complain: A familiar tightness under the shoulder blade returned after the last contraction. You begin kneading right over the spot, first with your fingertips and then with the whole hand. The room becomes quiet as people settle down for awhile to watch the

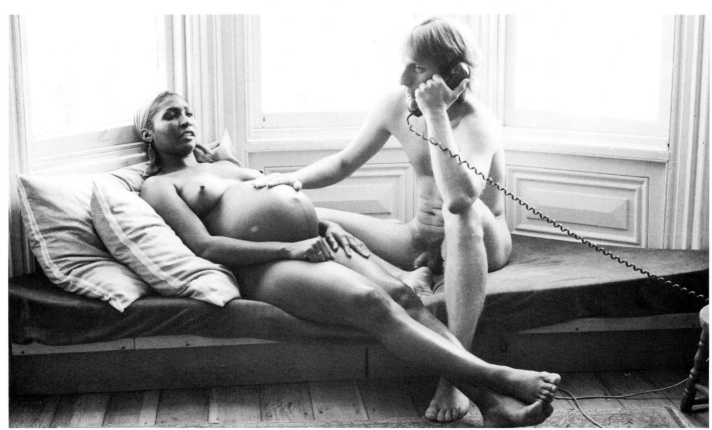

two of you. After a few minutes, when your kneading gives way to a friction sequence, you feel hardened muscles begin to soften. Pain and tension dissolve, leaving your partner relaxed and smiling.

Unless you're planning on delivering the baby personally, there will probably be other people in the delivery room while you massage. It may not always be possible for them to sit back, relax, and do nothing simply because births are unpredictable. Nevertheless, it helps to remind people that your partner will get more out of her massage in a quiet, peaceful atmosphere. By explaining how massage works, you're giving them "permission" to relax when they aren't involved in more important activities. Obviously, a delivery room that is crowded with anxious people who do nothing but rush around nervously will make a birth much more difficult. Given the chance to do some massage, you can make a real contribution to everyone's peace of mind and thereby help relax the mother-to-be. There is a ritual quality to massage, perhaps in the repetition of symmetrical movements, that quiets onlookers. They realize that silence, rather than fretful conversation, might serve a woman better between contractions, particularly when she is experiencing something as personal as massage.

If your partner is in the mood, soft, lyrical music (via radio or cassette) and some kind of pleasant scent can be added to the room. Don't abandon massage, however, if incense, music, and a relaxed atmosphere are not available. Your basic necessities—a squeeze bottle of oil and a soft towel—can be tucked into any delivery room no matter how much elaborate equipment is around. If you are in a hospital, try not to be intimidated by high-tech medical gadgets. Long before any of them were invented, men were massaging women in labor.

Your partner may request a specific stroke or ask that you concentrate on a certain spot. Just as often, though, a woman simply wants to feel your hands massaging her body, and selecting an area will be up to you. If she makes no particular request, begin massaging on the neck and shoulder area, and return to it often. Since this is one of the first places where stress-related muscle tension shows up in women, it's essential to keep it supple between contractions. See if you can begin with the side lying position, which is convenient for the neck and shoulders, but be flexible in case she needs to move around. If you're interrupted, wait for her to settle down again, and go back to what you were doing. Once you being massaging, the requests will usually come. Be ready with fast hand-over-hand circulation strokes if her hands or feet grow cold and with fingertip kneading for the whole limb.

There's no reason to stop massaging during labor pains; in fact, you may help alleviate the worst pain by continuing. Seventy-nine years ago, when massage was used routinely during the whole birth, Dr. Edgar F. Cyriax, a British medical researcher, observed that:

Frictions on the posterior sacral nerves (especially the third and fourth) and of the lumbar nerves, executed during each uterine pain, seem to aid materially in the expulsion of the foetus and afterwards of the placenta; they certainly diminish the pain in the back that is so often present, and make the patient feel more comfortable. *

At the very bottom of the spine you can feel the sacrum, a flat, roughly triangular bone where five vertebrae are neatly fused together (see illustration, page 111). The third and fourth sacral nerves that Dr. Cyriax got excited about emerge very close to the center of the triangle. Don't worry about pinpointing their location because the sacrum is small enough for you to cover the whole of it with the fingers of one hand. When it's convenient and comfortable for your partner, use fingertip friction movements on the very bottom of the spine, where nerves branch out to the legs. Massaging this spot can be particularly effective in calming a woman after a contraction. Nerves that supply the uterus also originate in the lowest part of the spine. During sacral friction movements, you'll have to be flexible with your anchor hand as your partner moves around, but the best place for it is at the very top of the buttocks. If you need to anchor above the sacrum, be careful not to press too hard on her kidneys. Choose a smooth rhythm with your friction hand that can be sustained for a long time if necessary.

Use massage during labor to relax a woman and offer her tangible support through the final contractions. When the Victorian Dr. Cyriax prudently

* E.F. Cyriax, *Elements of Kellgren's Manual Treatment,* (London: William Wood & Co., 1904), pp. 237–38.

recommended lower-back friction during "the expulsion of the foetus and afterwards of the placenta," he was referring to a process we now call, simply, the birth. Everything you've done with massage throughout pregnancy has been intended to facilitate this moment. Months of massage have added to tissues throughout the body a degree of suppleness that will now be put to the test. Bones, internal organs, tiny intervertebral ligaments and thick muscle bands that wrap halfway around the torso have been conditioned each time you massage.

well-meaning medical people. The twentieth-century delivery room is equipped for every contingency except perhaps the simple solution to a simple problem. Be ready, if you're called upon to do some massage, also to explain briefly how important the experience has been to your partner.

When it works, massage during labor or delivery requires more endurance than fancy technique from the masseur. Usually a woman will ask you to concentrate on one or two parts of her body—say, the shoulders and lower back. She may have a

To anchor sacral friction spread your thumb and forefinger and press down from above.

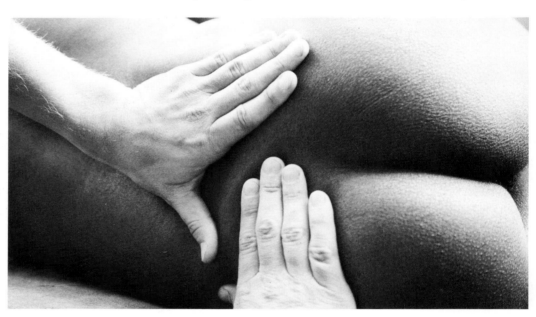

Fluid release strokes cleared irritating wastes from the muscles and kept them well supplied with important nutrients. Blood vessels of the legs that benefitted from deep circulation movements will more easily accept the pressures of an increased heart rate during delivery. Even nerve endings which were cleared of microscopic debris each time you massaged are less likely to become irritated.

In the late nineteenth century, before pain-killing drugs became popular, massage was used routinely by physicians and midwives during delivery. Today the physician has access to roomfuls of sophisticated equipment to help with the birth and deal with potential complications. Deliveries are unpredictable, of course, and a woman should have the benefit of every possible resource. Unfortunately the fact that massage can physically aid a mother during birth may meet with some resistance from

favorite movement, such as shoulder friction, to which you can add occasional hand-over-hand stroking, fingertip kneading, and circulation movements for variation. Be ready to continue for the better part of an hour if necessary. If you become fatigued, see if somebody else can take over while you rest. Team massage works well during labor because less experienced members of the team need learn only a few strokes to be effective (see Team Massage, page 66). Choose calm people for your team who will be content to copy a few basic movements without improvising.

AFTER THE BIRTH

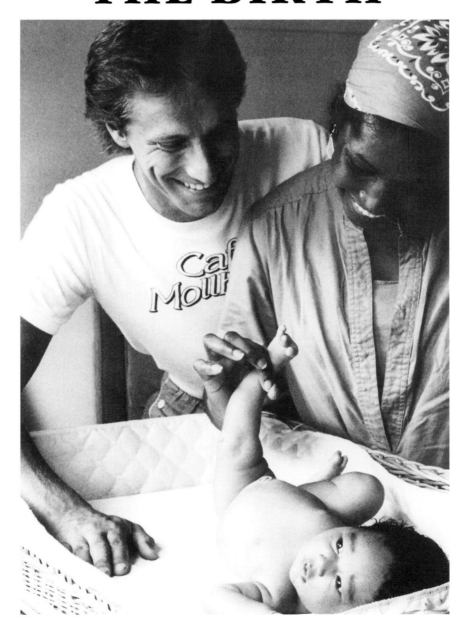

The First Month

Before I got married I had six theories about bringing up children,
now I have six children and no
theories.

Lord Rochester

After the birth begin massage with
simple movements that have
immediate results. Friction and
stroking movements around your
partner's shoulders will make it
possible for you to go on to the
lower back and abdomen or the
neck and head.

Exactly what sort of treatment should a woman
receive after birth? A casual look at the world's cul-
tures produces a bewildering variety of answers to
this question. Brazilian tribal women are at work in
the fields a few days after delivery, but new Chinese
mothers are encouraged to do nothing at all for an
entire month. During this period, literally called
"doing the month," they avoid sex, communal
meals, exposure to the wind, reading, crying, walking, and bathing. Nigerian women bathe three times
a day for six weeks and eat plenty of fish soup. To
strengthen and purify the body, the Indians of
northern Mexico become vegetarians, while the Tai-
wanese woman consumes nearly a whole chicken
daily. In various parts of the world the placenta is
buried, burned, enshrined, ignored, or eaten. Just
fifty years ago American women were encouraged
to embrace the idea of painless childbirth. The
modern mother gave birth while totally anesthe-
tized and then remained in bed, where she could be
closely observed, for several weeks. Women are
confined after birth in Egypt; worshipped in Poly-
nesia; and scorned (if they "pamper" themselves) in
certain parts of Ireland.

Proposing yet another approach to postpartum
care is outside the scope of this book, but whatever
method you choose, massage will be helpful. The
role of massage in the first few weeks after a birth is
to bring a couple together and help restore the
mother. Important physical and psychological benefits to a woman who is massaged after a birth have
been recognized throughout the world since biblical
times. In Malaysia, where specially trained practitioners called *tukang urut* begin massage immediately after birth, the women are known for their
lovely figures, which always seem to return after
childbirth. Similar practices were popular in the
West until doctors began using cost-effective drugs
instead of massage. Medical literature of the early
twentieth century is full of praise for massage cures
based on periodic friction and kneading sessions.

This is a time to look inside a woman for the
source of her feelings. Deal with postpartum stress,
pain, and fatigue in the tissues of her body. Take
your time, and let her feel how much you care.
Now, perhaps more than any other time in life, a

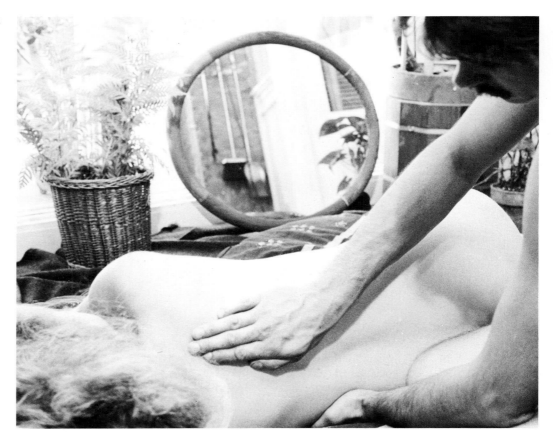

woman's thoughts and moods are directly related to physical events taking place within her.

Childbirth puts such a severe strain on abdominal muscles that permanent damage can result. After being stretched far beyond their normal length in the third trimester, the muscles are subjected to even more punishing strains during delivery. When the stretching is finally relieved after the birth, and exhaustion takes the place of tension, there is a very real danger that the overworked muscles will never regain any useful level of toning. That leaves a woman with a permanently flabby abdominal area with once-taut muscles now hanging in limp, fleshy folds. Unfortunately the problem is more than just cosmetic.

Well-toned abdominal muscles exert a continual light massaging action on the intestines during walking or running. Even if one remains perfectly still, the movement of the diaphragm during respiration will effectively flex the abdominal muscles. When the muscles lose their shape, the intestines are deprived of this internal massage, and frequent constipation is likely. Weakening of internal muscles can interfere with digestion until the absorption of food within the intestines is interrupted. Finally, circulation throughout the whole abdominal area, which is aided by frequently contracting muscles, becomes sluggish. As early as one month after childbirth, these degenerative changes can become terribly permanent and the source of constant problems to a new mother.

The best way to restore abdominal muscles to their original condition is through movement and massage. A certain amount of rest for the overworked muscular and nervous systems is necessary after childbirth. Each woman will have different requirements, but it is essential that she avoid yielding to fatigue and becoming a semi-invalid for weeks at a time. At some point, usually early on, exercise becomes far more therapeutic than bed rest, and a woman who wants to remain healthy should take advantage of every opportunity to move about. She can learn to balance the need for exercise against day-to-day changes in her physical condition.

During the postpartum period a masseur must carefully integrate his services with the bustling schedule of a new mother. Although this should be a peaceful time, new patients are often faced with unexpected problems that can seem much more important than daily massage. Well-meaning guests who want to see the new baby will advance on the new mother, requiring time, attention, and perhaps food. The authoritarian exercise therapist, a familiar figure in Victorian times, is likely to turn up, bristling with worrisome advice and unsolicited opinions. Dietitians, midwives, and psychologists are ready with tempting self-improvement programs that can occupy half an afternoon. It's important for new parents to schedule activities so that enough time is available each day for massage. Try to choose a time toward the end of the day close to your partner's bedtime and when the baby is likely to be asleep. If your new child suddenly needs attention during the massage, be prepared to return to what you were doing after he settles down.

Listen carefully to what your partner says about herself so you can modify each day's massage to her changing needs. Pay special attention to physical problems, such as cramping and fatigue, that will respond nicely to fluid release sequences. Elevated arterial blood pressure that usually prevails during the birth will drop rapidly to normal levels. If her extremities become temporarily chilled when this happens, you can use vigorous circulation strokes to ease the discomfort.

Deep stretch marks on the abdomen, like wrinkles on the face, are an indication of weakness in the underlying muscle structure. The skin is elastic enough to reshape itself once the muscles have been restored to full tone, and after the birth you have about three weeks to do something about overstretched muscles before they become a permanent problem. That's plenty of time to bring them back into shape with massage and a few basic exercises even when extra bed rest is required.* You can also use massage as an antidote to the depression caused by the overwhelming muscle and nerve fatigue that always follows a birth. Fifteen minutes of fluid release technique can be more effective in relieving postpartum depression than hours of psychological counseling.

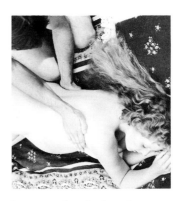

Pregnancy is a shock to the system and a great strain. Nevertheless, massage is effective against much more serious physical disruptions. When contusions, sprains and dislocations are massaged regularly the immediate symptoms disappear quickly. More serious consequences like wasting, weakness, contraction and stiffness are prevented.

---

*If your partner has had an episiotomy, consult with your doctor before beginning any exercise or massage program.

125

The First Through the Fourth Days

You can begin with massage the first day after delivery, when the muscles of the abdominal wall are still sore and painful. On the first and second days combine gentle abdominal strokes with deep breathing exercises to begin relaxing your partner and strengthening her overfatigued muscles. Deep breathing strengthens the diaphragm (the thick horizontal sheet of muscle that presses up on the lungs), oxygenates the blood, and accelerates the removal of gaseous wastes. Since all three benefits complement the fluid release effect, this simple exercise is a valuable aid to postpartum massage. Your partner may have had some difficulty with breathing exercises before the birth. Even though she's close to exhaustion now, be sure to encourage her to try again. Once the pressure from below the lungs has been relieved, deep breathing becomes a pleasant luxury instead of a chore.

Shallow breathing is limited to the upper chest, and the lungs are never filled to capacity. Deep breathing, however, combines tightening of the abdominal wall with complete oxygen combustion. Your partner sucks the air in through her nose by expanding her abdomen (thereby pulling down on the diaphragm) and pushes air out by sucking in her stomach. A woman should be able to watch her abdomen flatten and expand as she inhales and exhales slowly. Deep breathing can't be rushed, or your partner will begin to feel dizzy.

Once she has established a comfortable rhythm, you can help her get more out of the exercise by moving her arms in time with the breathing. Grasp her arms at the wrists, and raise them over her head as she inhales; then lower them to her waist as she exhales. This allows her rib cage to expand fully with each breath and then compress all the way during exhalation. Two dozen deep breaths are enough, in the beginning, to prepare a woman for postpartum massage. Over the next few weeks, as she gets stronger, she can do more breathing and you can add more massage.

Begin with a heart-shaped stroking movement just below the center of the lowest ribs. Follow the ribs outward to the side of her body, and then turn your hands inward, stroking along the abdomen, until they meet over the navel. From there, bring your hands straight up until they reach the starting position below the ribs. As you repeat this stroke, the lowest point of the movement should descend gradually until your hands are traveling across the bottom of the abdomen.

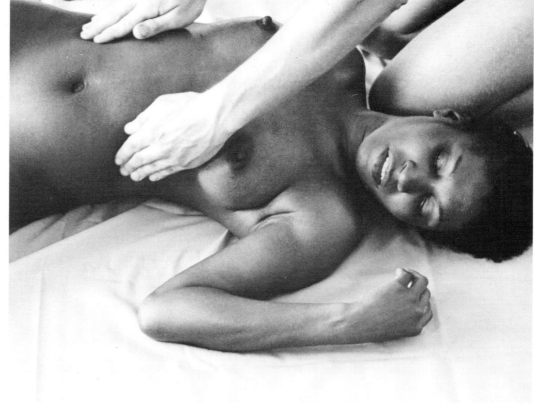

When massaging your partner's abdomen on the first day after delivery, you can use more pressure than you have in months. Use pillows to elevate her knees until they are high enough to relax the muscles of the abdomen. A woman will usually experience considerable relief after only a few minutes of stroking the abdomen. As she relaxes, you can begin a series of deeper kneading strokes across the whole of her abdomen. Follow this with light frictions across the top and up and down the sides of the abdomen to stimulate the colon and prevent possible constipation. Fifteen minutes of massage on each of the first two days will usually relieve abdominal pain while stimulating circulation and toning stretched-out muscles. This is a particularly important time to encourage feedback from your partner so you know exactly how you're doing. Be ready to give extra attention to unexpected problems like leg cramps or a headache.

On the third and fourth days repeat everything you did on the first two days, and add a general massage of all four limbs. Begin and end with a long circulation movement on each limb to stimulate circulation and clear the lymphatic system. The deep breathing exercises should be performed more vigorously.

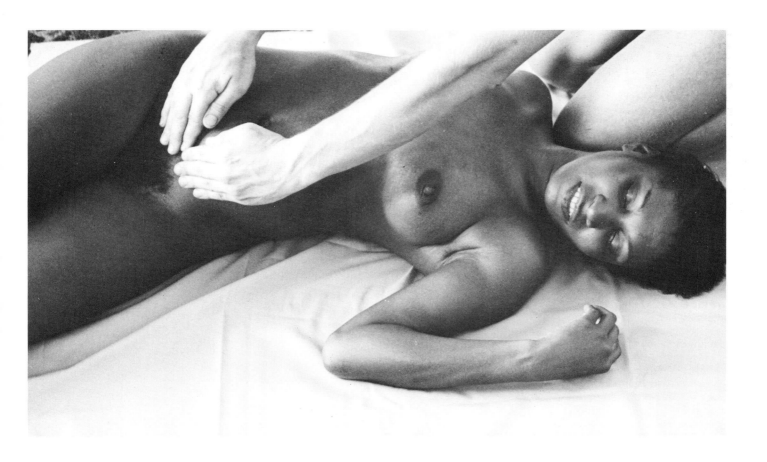

The Fifth to the Ninth Days

Individuals calling themselves "pressure point masseurs" insist that the body is covered with mysterious little buttons that make magical things happen whenever they are pushed. While various teachers argue about where the buttons are located their enthusiastic students jab away self-righteously at the softest parts of defenseless "patients."

One esoteric theory follows another: acupuncture, which requires years of medical training, has been replaced by "the accupressure weekend" and finally by something called "Accu-yoga." We know that ginseng is beneficial but must we now use ginseng toothpaste?

The notion that the body is a spooky place that must be tortured back to good health was even more popular during the sexually repressive Victorian age than it is now. Turning human beings into a supernatural puzzle satisfies the reactionary puritan because it takes us further away from the natural body. Real massage, however, offers a revolutionary approach to the body: that pleasure itself is therapeutic.

Douglas Graham, the great 19th century American physician-masseur, used these pictures to ridicule "therapists" who attempted to substitute pressure points for massage. Direct pressure to a blood vessel will cut off circulation and, eventually, cause local muscles to cramp. Pain causes the muscles to tense up and go into spasm. Nevertheless, short cut therapies are still popular and just as futile as they were a hundred years ago.

By the fifth day your partner can begin a series of exercises that combine leg lifts with abdominal tightening during extended deep breathing. All these exercises can be performed in bed if she's still feeling weak. Their main purpose is to strengthen the abdominal muscles, which can now be put under mild strain without danger. You can help your partner get started by having her draw up a knee during inhalation and extend it as she exhales. On the extension movement, her leg should descend to a perfectly flat position. She can emphasize the last part of the exhalation by pointing her toes forward as the leg is extended. After twenty-five repetitions of this movement place a pillow under the knees, and assist her with deep breathing by raising and lowering her arms in rhythm as she inhales and exhales.

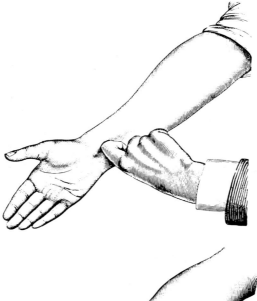

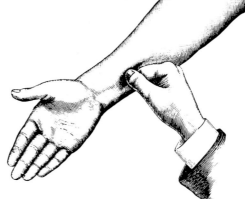

You are now tightening the abdominal muscles from above as well as from below. After a few minutes of breathing exercises flex her knees, and begin to massage the abdomen and limbs. Hand-over-hand circulation strokes on the thighs will help promote good circulation throughout the abdomen as well as in the legs. Once you've done twenty on each thigh, elevate her knees, and return to the abdomen for fingertip kneading strokes. Keeping the abdom-prevent muscle collapse that leads to permanent stretch marks.

This marks the beginning of your active role as masseur in the three-week critical recovery period of overstretched abdominal muscles. Patient repetition of ordinary kneading movements will restore their tone and sometimes erase the last visible signs of pregnancy.

By the end of the first week, provided there have been no unusual complications, it's time to work on the stretched, and probably weakened, muscles in the perineal region. A good way to begin strengthening them is through a series of resistive exercises, consisting of pressing movements made by your partner against resistance supplied by you.

With one knee drawn up against her chest (or as high as it will go comfortably), your partner pushes up on her whole leg while you push down, holding it in place. This shouldn't turn into a struggle but rather can be an informal balancing of force between the two of you. Hold the leg in a permanently flexed position while she presses up to extend it. If she can manage to contract the muscles of the perineal region at the same time, the exercises will have an even more beneficial effect.

If a woman experienced a normal vaginal birth without episiotomy, she should now be ready for a more vigorous leg and abdominal exercise program. (Again, consult your doctor after an episiotomy to find out when it's safe to begin these more strenuous exercises.) You can continue helping with resistive exercises for the perineal muscles and add trunk lifts near the sacrum. By this time she will also want to begin unassisted leg lifts and thigh stretching. You can extend your massage to any part of the body that seems sore (that is, if surgery was not performed). Remember to avoid deep pressure strokes on the inner thigh, where they will interfere with arterial circulation. Use pillows to keep your partner comfortable, and try 100 identical circulation strokes on the back. She has come through lots of pain; now you can substitute continuous pleasure.

Blood pressure and volume levels are finally returning to normal. During the transition period coldness or numb feelings in the extremities will usually disappear after a few minutes of fingertip kneading and stroking toward the heart.

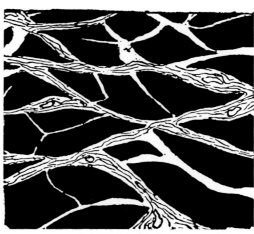

WITHOUT MASSAGE

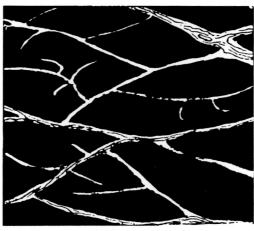

AFTER REGULAR MASSAGE

Inside the muscles before and after massage: After massage the intermuscular tissue is firm and well defined. Without massage the intermuscular tissue is thickened while the muscle bundles are thinner and compressed.

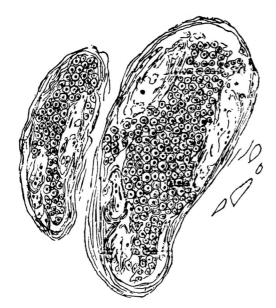

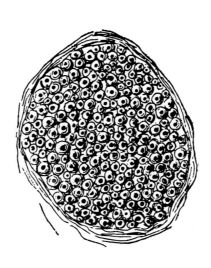

Inside the nerves before and after massage: After massage the nerve elements have been cleansed of microscopic debris and appear whole and uncrowded. They are held together by a thin bundle of connective tissue that forms the outer sheath. Without massage the sheath becomes thickened and underneath it layers of connective tissue crowd the nerve fibers. Nerve debris, that interferes with electrical transmission, is evident.

WITHOUT MASSAGE   AFTER REGULAR MASSAGE

This is the time to begin experimenting with exercises that involve lifting and stretching large parts of the body. You can help with leg and pelvic lifts until a woman feels comfortable doing them alone. Abdominal or pelvic lifts coupled with deep breathing will begin strengthening the crucial stomach muscles you've been massaging for the past two weeks. Whole leg lifts and sit-ups are much more difficult, but they shouldn't be ruled out. Both exercises can be incorporated gradually.

Mother and father now face a new set of responsibilities as parents, and that realization can produce frightening tensions. What better way to begin resolving them than with an *exchange* of massage? It may take hours or days to talk out your differences, but it takes only a few minutes to relax the muscles of the neck and shoulders and pump fresh oxygen into the brain. Massage may help both of you think clearly and plan for the days to come.

The same strokes that are effective on a woman will work on a man. Men tend to accumulate tension in the muscles of the lower back and calves rather than in the neck and shoulders. Shared massages should be at least a few hours apart if only to allow the massaged person to relax afterward. A father who feels shut out by the new mother will get the attention he deserves during a twenty-minute back massage. If he seems testy and nervous, give him a massage instead of an argument, and you may see the tension between the two of you vanish.

Very few men have actually experienced a real massage. Ask him what he wants and he'll usually ask for a back rub. Happily, you can easily do much more for a new father than merely rubbing his back. Start by relaxing the whole lower back and for the next massage extend the feeling of relaxation and pleasure to the hands, arms, legs and feet.

Once your partner is warm and comfortable you may notice that he seems nervous about being massaged. Most men are not accustomed to simply surrendering to physical pleasure. Let him know that you're going to do all the work during the massage and there will be no demands on him. Concentrate, at first, on simply feeling him breathe. Let your hands rise and fall gently on the surface of his back. This simple act of caring takes both of you one step closer to a completely relaxed mood.

Concentrate on building a hypnotic mood if your primary concern is relaxation. Start with a slow easy rhythm when you begin massaging and try to stay with it. Be sure your partner doesn't feel obligated to correct your technique. Practice sessions can occur at a different time. A few words

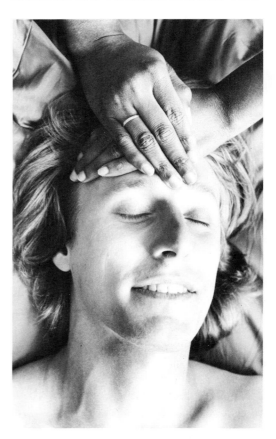

of feedback are O.K. but don't encourage conversation. Always keep some part of your body touching his. This gives continuity to your massage and encourages him to experience sensation with every part of his body.

If it's your first time massaging you may feel nervous. You don't need to be, though, because it's going to work. Even though your technique may not be perfect your partner will enjoy *being touched*. Stick with movements that you know well and repeat them many times.

A woman can begin to strengthen her stomach muscles by lifting a single knee, raising her head with both hands or lifting just the head and shoulders, instead of the whole torso. Once the sit-up and whole leg lift have become fluid, you have a good indication that she's close to full recovery.

To the new mother:
If your partner's been under a lot of pressure he's likely to fall asleep while you're massaging. Don't feel that you've failed as a masseuse if this happens. You've succeeded in releasing accumulated tension from his body without resorting to a drug. Massage induced sleep is deep and satisfying. He'll awake feeling refreshed, energized and very grateful.

Massaging the Breasts during Lactation

Any woman who is breast-feeding has learned to express—to start the milk flowing without the baby's help. This simple process, one of the few times where self-massage has any real value, will come into frequent use during breast-feeding. When, for various reasons, a woman cannot get her breasts to express, you can usually help with massage movements that amplify the expressing effect.

If the breasts are simply overfull, cover them with a light sweet oil (like almond) and begin stroking very gently, the same way she did, from

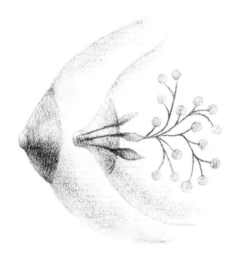

the periphery to the nipple. Help her with the first part of expressing, the stroking, and let her finish by herself. Cup the breast with one hand, and stroke down toward the areola with the other. Keep your fingers together, and allow your stroking hand to shape itself to the contour of her breast. Stroke down only as far as the edge of the areola. This is an especially important time to encourage feedback from your partner and determine exactly what she's feeling.

Remember the location of sensitive areas, and as they return to normal while you're massaging, go back and massage them again with light friction movements. Give her plenty of light stroking with fingertip kneading and selective light friction for variation. After a few minutes sit back, relax, and let her try to express the breast(s) once again. You will usually see happy results very quickly.

Occasionally the breasts will fail to express because local blood and lymph vessels are so full that the flow of milk is temporarily blocked. Although this condition is not serious it feels much more uncomfortable than ordinary milk engorgement. A few minutes of conversation will help both of you identify the problem and send it on its way. Techniques that were useful in stimulating milk flow will only force more blood into the breasts, worsening an already uncomfortable situation. Usually, a woman will get relief by simply bathing her breasts in very warm water until they either begin leaking milk spontaneously or the "self-massage" sequence for expressing milk succeeds. You can sometimes help relieve the pressure by stroking away from the periphery of the breasts in the direction of major blood vessels. Stay off the breasts themselves and use light pressures, which can increase gradually. Some women will benefit from a series of short hand-over-hand stroking movements that begin just above the breast and press out towards the shoulders.

Pay special attention to a woman who experiences intense pain when lactation becomes erratic. Unusual breast pain deserves prompt medical attention. In this case, before you demonstrate how effective massage is at moving fluids around inside the body, ask a physician which way they need to be moved. If the breasts are infected, massage may spread the infection to other parts of the body.

Worry and anxiety will also interfere with breast feeding. If that becomes a persistent problem you may need to massage the whole woman and let her breasts take care of themselves.

Expressing milk is a two-part operation for a woman. She begins by stroking down the top surface of her breast with one hand while cupping it with the other. Once she has stroked the whole top of the breast, stimulated the milk glands, and moved milk down toward the nipple, she squeezes the edge of the areola (not the nipple itself) until milk squirts out in a tiny jet.

SPECIALIZED MASSAGE

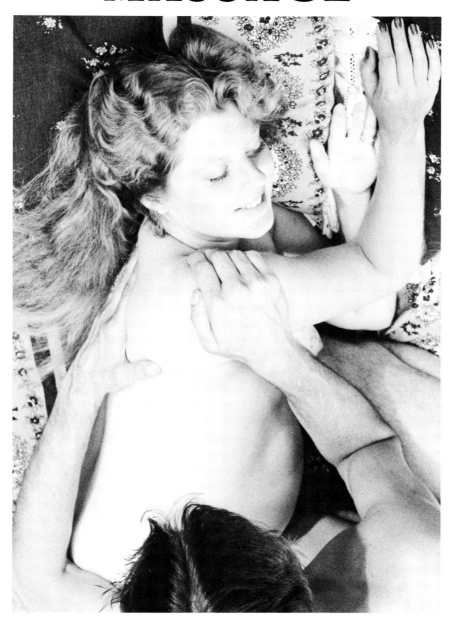

Massage as Therapy

Our modern mother-to-be sits alone in a furnished room surrounded by how-to-have-a-baby and what-to-do-with-children books, each volume more self-assured and strident than the last. Outside, it's raining, so a walk is not a very good idea. Where would she go anyway? She doesn't feel fashionable or self-assured, and she hasn't had a positive thought in weeks.

Her man enters the room, but he seems far away and out of touch. He sits down nearby without speaking, takes her hand, and the two of them feel her abdomen. Perhaps that moment isn't covered in the strident self-help books because it can't be planned or easily defined. One is finally alone with a growing creature, already as alive as you are and ready to take a turn at life in this world.

For husband and wife the unpredictable psychological changes that accompany pregnancy can be terrifying. Rapid mood shifts caused by accelerated hormonal activity are confusing, and of course, the new role of parent with its awesome responsibilities can badly frighten either partner. Great intensity is always difficult to sustain or control, and what could possibly be more intense than creation itself?

The question is: How can you use massage to support a pregnant woman when she's depressed? Massage can influence many of her mood shifts because they are caused by internal conditions. Accumulated acidic wastes in the muscles leave a woman exhausted, but an even more important mood-altering factor is the effect of poor circulation on body temperatures. It may be useful to consider the massage solution to this problem the next time your pregnant partner becomes unexpectedly depressed.

[The baby] can feel the snug embrace of the uterine walls, the heat of the mother's body and hear the pounding rhythm of her heartbeat, thumping away at 72 beats per minute. These are the primary impressions of human life on earth, and they make a lasting impact . . .

When the baby is born it experiences a sudden loss of these vital signals.

Desmond Morris

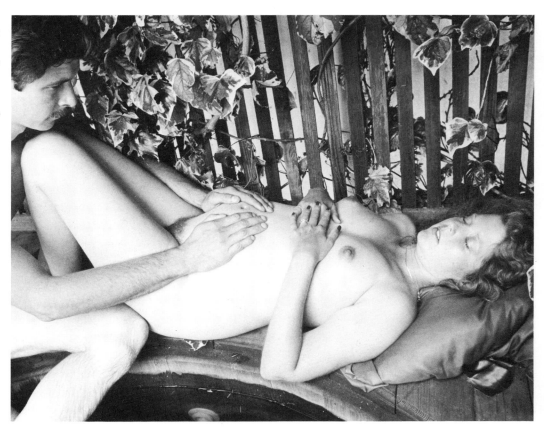

The temperature functions of the body, which control the production, dissipation, and regulation of heat, are so intimately connected to a person's mood that an internal variation of just a few tenths of a degree at the wrong time of the day is enough to cause sudden depression. Once again, what appears to be an intractable mental problem merely represents a temporary physical distraction, and a few minutes of massage will usually restore your partner's good spirits. Normally body temperature will fluctuate by as much as two degrees Fahrenheit over a twenty-four-hour period. Maximum temperatures occur around 2:00 P.M., when circulation is the most vigorous throughout the body. Not surprisingly this is the most productive part of the workday. Minimum body temperature comes at 2:00 A.M., when the heart slows down and most people are asleep. This temperature variation pattern is so automatic that people will cling to it stubbornly even though work hours and other responsibilities may change. Trouble begins when well-established heat regulation patterns are overruled by the new demands of pregnancy. Increased blood volume,

heart size, and body weight strain the circulatory system and sometimes restrict blood flow while the body adapts to new conditions. Grumpiness at the breakfast table may be not bad manners or hormonal changes but low temperature.

If your partner's skin feels cool to the touch, concentrate on deep kneading strokes, which will raise the temperature of large muscles almost immediately. Superficial friction strokes are useful when the skin feels warm (but not feverish). After a few minutes of repetition the heat dissipation rate from the surface of the body will double, and she should feel relieved and cooler. These are temporary effects, however, and it's far more important to use massage on a daily basis to promote normal heat regulation through good circulation. As strenuous exercise becomes difficult, a pregnant woman may come to depend on regular massage to keep her circulation brisk and her spirits up.

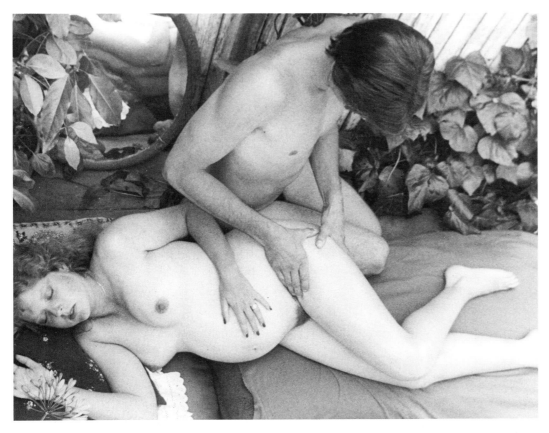

A newly born child immediately craves the warmth and contact of the womb. A mother's embrace reminds the child of the world he has just left. So does a few minutes of body massage.

Drugs or Massage?

The important physical and psychological advantages a woman can gain from massage are seriously compromised by addictive drugs. Unfortunately the addictive personality is a very real phenomenon, and addiction to one drug usually means involvement with many. How much influence can massage have on any body system if it must compete with substances that set the heart pounding as adrenaline is pumped into the veins while blood sugar levels plummet and soar? The real issue for a pregnant woman is control of her body and the body of her growing child.

If drugs isolate people, massage brings them together. You remain in physical contact with your partner throughout a massage. Even when you're not actively massaging, you're touching because to stop touching, even for a moment, leaves your partner feeling alone and abandoned. Every moment something is shared.

Massage is a powerful tool that will provide you with drug-free solutions to many of the physical and psychological problems in pregnancy. An ener-

The Finns move in less than a few seconds from a heat of 170F to a cold of -50F, which makes a difference of more than 220 degrees, and the effect is very much the same as if they jumped from boiling into freezing water.

In the sauna, they say, they regain their strength far more quickly than when they rest or sleep. The hot steam softens their skin to such an extent that they can shave without soap and with the very worst of razors.

A complaint is made that women often give birth to their children in the sauna. Finnish doctors have in fact found recently that the custom of Saturday bathing tends to encourage the onset of labor, with a disproportionate number of Finnish babies being born on Monday.

H.J. Viherjuuri

Drugs That Cross the Placental Barrier and May Endanger the Fetus

Drug	Adverse effect
Acetaminophen (Excedrin, Datril, Tylenol, Sinutab, Vanquish, and others)	Methemoglubinemia (a cyanotic condition often resulting in a bluish discoloration because of an excessive concentration of reduced hemoglobin in the blood)
Ammonium chloride (Benylin Cough Syrup, Coricidin Cough Relief Formula, and others)	Acidosis (a pathological condition characterized by an accumulation of acid in the body)
Androgens (Formatrix)	Congenital heart defects, limb reduction effects, increased risk of vaginal or cervical cancer in later life, and other serious effects
Aspirin (salicylates)	Ulcers and hemmorrhaging in mother; bleeding in newborn infant and possible severe hypoglycemia
Barbiturates (Donnatal, Nembutal, Belap, Donphen, Plexonal, Seconal Amytal, Butisol, and others)	Depressed respiration
Amphetamines (Dexedrine)	Possible malformation of the great blood vessels of the heart
Bishydroxycoumarin (Dicumerol)	Fetal death and internal hemorrhage
Chloral hydrate (Aquachloral Suprettes, Felsules capsules, Noctec, and others) in large doses	Fetal death
Chloramphenicol (Chloramphenicol Capsules, Chloromycetin Kapseals and Capsules, and others)	Fetal death
Chloropromazine (Chloropromazine Hydrochloride Tablets, Chloropromazine HCL VSP Tablets, Thorazine)	Neonatal jaundice, possible fetal death, or abnormalities of the brain
Chlorpropamide (Diabenese)	Prolonged neonatal hypoglycemia (lowered blood sugar)
Cortisone	Cleft palate
Heroin	Neonatal addiction, death and respiratory depression
Iodides (Elioxphylin, Isoprel Compound, Pediocof, Theokin Elixir and Tablets, Calcidrine Syrup, Ephed Organdin Tablets and Elixir, Pima Syrup, and others)	Goiter

getic masseur who is generous enough to sacrifice half an hour of sleep to put somebody else to sleep can eliminate most but not all over-the-counter drugs.

Determining which medicinal drugs can be taken safely during pregnancy becomes more confusing as more new drugs appear each year. Thalidomide has demonstrated to the world just how dangerous new drugs can be for a pregnant woman. Nevertheless, certain drugs, if not the very newest ones, will usually be helpful at some point.

Part of the educational process for couples who are committed to massage is learning exactly how far they can go without drugs. Some fortunate women can go all the way to the birth. More commonly, however, a woman will eventually encounter pain that doesn't respond to friction or a headache that stubbornly hangs on after a two-minute forehead press. If you have seen massage work wonders, don't be discouraged when your partner takes a pill—massage will work again, and the next time you may not need the pill. And when you find

Drug	Adverse effect
Isoniazid (INH Tablets, Nydraeid Injection/ Tablets/Syrup, Rifamate, Rimactagid, and others)	Retarded psychomotor activity
Leorophanol (Levo-Dromoran)	Fetal respiratory depression
Lithium carbonate (Eskalith, Lithane, Lithium Carbonate Capsules and Tablets, Lithonate, Lithotabs)	Fetal respiratory depression
Lysergic acid diethylamide (LSD)	Chromosomal damage, stunted offspring
Ethanol (Beer, wine, whiskey, and others)	Fetal death, fetal alcohol syndrome, hyperactivity
Mepivacaine (Carbocaine Hydrochloride)	Slowing of fetal heart beat and neonatal depression
Methadone	Fetal respiratory depression
Methaqualine (Quaalude, Sopor)	Produces physical defects in developing embryo
Morphine	Newborn addicted and at risk of respiratory depression
Nicotine (cigarettes)	Low birthweight, elevated infant mortality
Phenmetrazine (Preludin)	Congenital abnormalities
Phenobarbital	Hemorrhage and death of newborn infant
Quinine	Deafness, decreases in number of blood platelets in infant
Resperine	Nasal block
Streptomycin	Hearing loss and abnormal shortness of arms or legs, damage to important nerves in head
Sulfanomides (long acting)	Destructive changes in nerves; atrophy of liver, anemia
Tetracycline	Discolored teeth, abnormal shortness of arms or legs, webbed hands
Thiazides (Diuril, Diapres, Aldoclor Tablets, Aquatensen, Enduron)	Neonatal death, decrease in blood platelets

Drugs or Massage? continued

yourself combining massage and drugs, remember that massage accelerates circulation and boosts internal nutrition. Consequently, most drugs will take effect faster and often with greater intensity. The notion that *every* drug or chemical is unsafe during pregnancy is a recipe for everlasting jitters. A woman can spend nine months constantly fiddling with her body, nervously scrutinizing the environment for "chemicals" (water is a chemical), and be tortured with guilt whenever she eats food from a strange kitchen. Or she can use common sense, avoid the obvious dangers, and relax. Here are some of the obvious dangers:

Common Medications Containing Nonrecommended Ingredients

Salicylates

Alka Seltzer	Comeback	Measurin*
Anacin	Cope	Midol
APC	Ecotrin*	Pamprin
ASA Compound	Empirin	Pyra-Gesic
Ascriptin	Compound	Salicorbate
Aspergum*	Excedrin	St. Joseph*
Bayer Aspirin*	Femicin	Trigesic
Bufferin	Liquiprin*	Vanquish

Para-aminophenol Derivatives: Phenacetin, Acetonalid, Acetaminophen

APC	Empirin	PAC
ASA Compound	Compound	Pamprin
Bromo-Seltzer	Excedrin	Percogesic
Comeback	Febrinol	Pyra-Gesic
Contramal	Tablets*	Tempra*
Compound	Femicin	Trendar
Counterpain	Medache	Trigesic
Datril*	Monthly Ets*	Tylenol*
	Nebs*	Vanquish
	Nilprin 7 ½ *	

CNS Stimulants: Xanthines

Anacin	Comeback	Femicin
APC	Cope	Midol
ASA Compound	Easy-Mens	Pre-Mens
Bromo-Seltzer	Empirin	Pyra-Gesic
	Compound	Trigesic
	Excedrin	Vanquish

*Drug contains one ingredient.

Data sources: E. W. Martin, *Hazards of Medication: A Manual on Drug Interactions, Incompatibilities, Contraindications, and Adverse Effects* (Philadelphia: J.B. Lippincott Co., 1978); Barbara Huff et al, (eds.) *Physicians Desk Reference,* 39th Edition (Oradell, New Jersey: Charles E. Baker, 1979).

Massaging Infants

Every baby loves to be touched and will enjoy simple massage a few days after birth. You may decide to include massage as part of after-bath drying and oiling or simply set aside some time when the child is relaxed and quiet. It's always fun for the father to get involved and show his new baby that both parents can be a source of pleasurable physical sensations. Once again, massage gives the father a more clearly defined role.

You can create a miniature circulation stroke by grasping the end of a limb just above the hand or foot, circling it with the thumb and forefinger of your other hand and stroking down to the torso. Flat hand stroking movements work well on the length of the torso and back, but you must be content to make contact with half a hand when the baby is very small. Abdominal kneading may be helpful if gas or constipation has been a problem and repetitive back stroking will often calm a nervous child. Light friction awakens the bottom of the feet and will stimulate circulation.

Be patient when you're interrupted and return to massage when the infant settles down. Forget about the methodical approach used on adults. You may find yourself pressing into the bottom of the feet one moment and on the back of the neck the next. Full body leaps are delightfully easy when massaging infants and a few quick fingertip kneading strokes on the first available flat surface will usually win a radiant smile. Fingertip kneading strokes, in fact, are the most universally effective movement for infant massage. The baby's entire torso may be only the thickness of an adult limb and the same fingertip kneading strokes that worked on the limb will be effective here. Wrap four fingers of each hand around the side of the torso and use the surface of your thumbs to first knead the back—then the stomach and rib cage.

People become easier to massage as they grow larger. Although infants love massage and will benefit from it just as much as adults, some strokes are limited by the size relationship between your hands and a part of the baby's body. Try to limit friction movements to the very tips of your fingers and hold off on percussion during the first few months.

How pleasant it would be, if in another state of being we could have shapes like our former selves for playthings, we standing outside or inside of them, as we liked, and they being to us just what we used to be to others!

Oliver Wendell Holmes

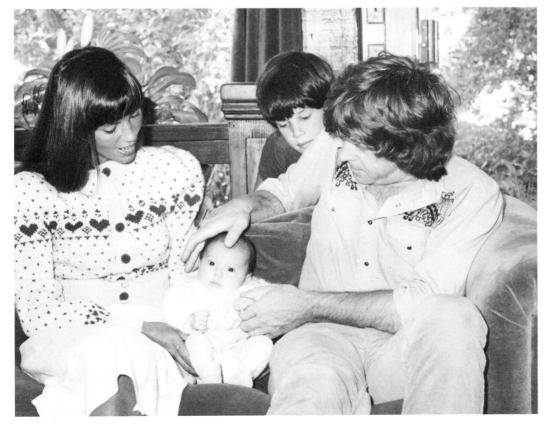

Along with the many physical benefits massage offers an infant, there is a vital psychological one. Modern psychologists have commented on the way people who are deprived of physical contact during childhood become cold, unfeeling individuals later on in life. Massage keeps you physically involved with a child and provides a good reason to spend time just touching him. During the playful physical bonding between mother and child immediately after birth, your baby learns that the world is a friendly place full of warm feelings. Use massage to carry that lesson into the future.

9

Massage Toys and Resources

The basic requirements for massage are a comfortable quiet place and a bottle of warm vegetable oil. If you live in a cold climate or a noisy environment the following chart may be helpful in creating the right atmosphere. A few minutes preparing your massage area will eliminate potential problems and increase your partner's pleasure. Professional masseurs and advanced amateurs who like to dabble with exotic special effects are invited to consider the chart the next time they shop for new toys. Have fun but remember that people have been massaging each other for thousands of years without high speed electrical devices.

The most important accessory for any masseur (and one that has survived in the ruins of ancient civilizations) is the massage table. A good one eliminates the strain of working on the floor, you work at waist level, and makes it easy to massage for the better part of an evening. Try that on your next special occasion and your partner will feel the difference for several days and nights.

Massage Toys and Resources

Device	Use	Advantage
A permanent massage table	Provides an ideal massage surface	Eliminates bending at the waist
A portable massage table	Provides an ideal massage surface in any setting	Eliminates bending at the waist, can be set up anywhere, folds for easy handling
Quartz electric heaters	Heats your massage area	Silent, portable, fast
Tape recorder with auto reverse	Provides continuous music	Create or record your own massage music
Record turntable with "repeat" function	Provides continuous music	Turn your favorite record into massage music
Dimmer switch	Creates a pleasant low light in any room	Eliminates special lighting devices
Scented candles	Provides soft light and pleasing scent	Creates suitable massage atmosphere in any room
Incense	Scents your massage area	Works from a remote position, good for large areas
An electric vibrator	Scalp and limbs	Scalp massage without oil, very fast
Massage School	Become a professional masseur.	Learn to give pleasure with your hands, you will never be replaced by a machine

The table shown here, designed by David Mohrmann, can be built in a single afternoon using just a hammer and nails. Have a lumberyard pre-cut the wood to size and pick up some paint or stain if you want a finish. The completed table will be fairly heavy and difficult for one person to move. Nevertheless, wheels are not recommended simply because you don't want your partner rolling off during a massage. Make the table surface (without foam rubber) 6 inches below the masseur's waist. It should be long enough to accommodate your partner's entire body. A 76 inch table will satisfy almost anyone you will ever massage.

Above all, a massage table must be sturdy. Use 1 ½ inch nails or screws throughout. Rounding off sharp angles makes the table attractive and more pleasant to use. This optional extra step requires sandpaper and a little bit of muscle power. Use the lower shelf for towels, extra oil, alcohol and an electric vibrator. When you're not massaging the foam pad can be removed and your table becomes a useful, if slightly unusual, piece of furniture.

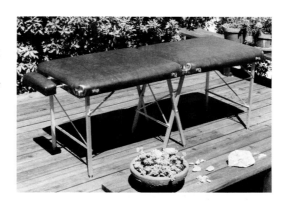

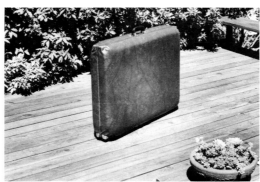

A good portable massage table comes with legs that adjust to several different levels. This helpful feature allows different sized people to massage each other on a single table. The headrest will support a woman's forehead during early pregnancy if she finds it difficult to turn her head to one side. Both the legs and headrest fit inside the folded table.

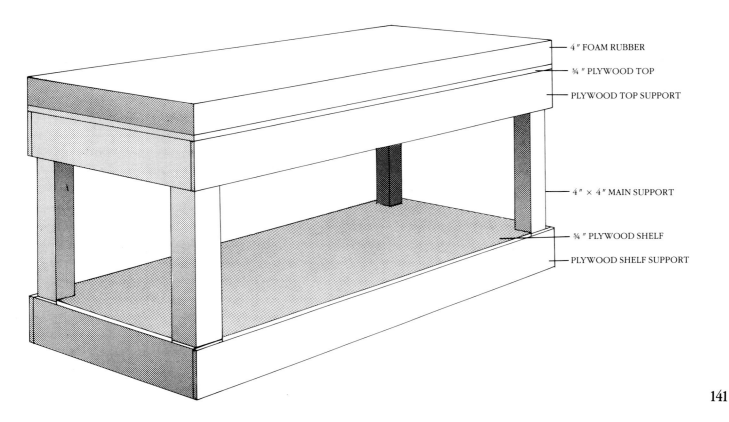

4″ FOAM RUBBER

¾″ PLYWOOD TOP

PLYWOOD TOP SUPPORT

4″ × 4″ MAIN SUPPORT

¾″ PLYWOOD SHELF

PLYWOOD SHELF SUPPORT

Shopping for a Professional Massage

A good masseur, like a good waiter, will attend to your needs and remain invisible. The very best masseur can study your body for a host of non-verbal "clues" and give you exactly what you need. Developing this kind of sensitivity may require a few sessions with gentle feedback from you. Don't be afraid to ask for whatever it is that you want. You know which shoulder needs more work, which muscles still feel sore, and what feels so good you don't want it to stop. Your concerns can be specific and very personal. Think about things that another person might not notice, and leave it to your masseur to remember to massage your left foot after finishing your left leg. Just as a waiter deserves to finish the evening washing dishes if he fails to bring you a cherished dessert, a masseur who actually skips a foot should be put to work in a hand laundry.

Lying down naked, with your eyes closed, on a massage table is an act of trust that is rare between strangers. A good masseur will reward you with an hour or two of uninterrupted physical pleasure. Still, there are "therapists" calling themselves masseurs who torture their clients in the name of some bizarre health theory (which has usually not been adequately translated into English). Beware of rolfers, deep zone therapists, shiatsu practitioners, and anyone else who promises a quick fix after certain mysterious points on your body have been poked while you limbs are being twisted into hazardous positions. It might be useful to discuss this concept with a new masseur before you begin so you'll know just what to expect. Don't be intimidated by puritanical "justifications" for pain or wall charts with lots of Chinese characters. One moment of pain will shatter an hour of tranquility. You shouldn't endure *anything* unpleasant during a massage.

A good massage, like a good meal, will make you feel wonderful while it's going on and for some time afterward. Nothing else matters more, and shoppers should be particularly wary of the masseur who promises satisfaction only after the fourth or fifth visit. Sensitivity is far more important than physical strength in massage, so you shouldn't be afraid to ask for lots of repetition if that's what you want. After the first few massages there's no reason to do a lot of talking during a session. You have a right to privacy simply because concepts and words will take your mind away from the feeling. A masseur who insists on conversation is defeating his own best efforts. If he doesn't comprehend your desires after a few sessions, it may be time to move on to somebody else.

Spend some time on the massage surface before the massage begins to be absolutely sure the area is warm enough for you. Ask for more heat if you feel the slightest chill; it will get worse as your metabolism slows and can ruin the massage. You might want to request a favorite oil or musical selection. Try not to schedule appointments immediately after a massage. A good masseur will create a warm, penetrating feeling that will last for hours. Let the feeling go on.

As we enter the speedy computer age and stress levels climb there has been a renewed interest in massage. Nearly every town has its licensed professional with a small group of devoted customers. Most professional masseurs work for themselves and have the satisfaction of knowing that every minute on the job something tangible and real is accomplished.